Ride On!

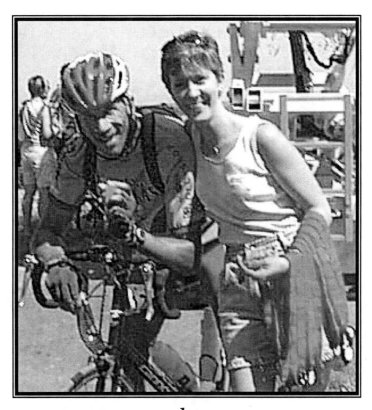

by

Stephanie M. Saulet

Booklocker.com, Inc.
2012

Linda,

Ride Majestically!

Ride Triumphantly!

Ride On the side of Truth!

Ride On for the Righteous Meek!

Psalm 45:4

Message Bible

Ride On strong in your faith, hope, and love through it all. (1 COR 13:7-8)

Stephanie

For Mark, Patrick, and Michael

"He who loves his brother remains in the light

and nothing in him will make him fall."

1ˢᵗ John 2:10

In loving honor and memory of

Christopher Nicolas Saulet

"If we love one another, God lives in us and

His love is made perfect for us."

1st John 4:12

Acknowledgments

With love and gratitude, I would like to acknowledge the following for their support throughout our fight and for cheering me on from the starting line to the finish line as I wrote this memoir.

God – *I strongly felt I was called to share our story. Being completely out of my comfort zone, I depended on Him to help me in the writing process. Through my prayers and time I've spent with God, I truly believe He led me through our story with His Words so that I could share them with you. He has shown me the many ways how His love prevails.*

Chris' brothers: Mark, Patrick, and Michael – *I'm blessed to have witnessed the special bond you shared together. Let your brotherly love continue.*

Our best friends: Bob and Kelly Schoonover – *For your special friendship and love. If it weren't for you, Chris and I would have never met and that would have been a tragedy for all of us.*

My parents, Bill and Helen DuFour – *Thank you for loving me so much to adopt me and giving me a family. I know you'll always be watching over me. I love you mom and dad.*

My sister, Carol Al-Kobri – *For all the times you've been there for me in ways only a sister can.*

My family – *For standing by my side in all that I've done and been through in my life.*

Teddie Fitzpatrick (AKA Teddie Momma) – *My mentor and dear friend. You taught me how to grow deeper in my faith. You were there for Chris and me, always prayerful and always hopeful. And you still are.*

Bob and Sue Schoonover (AKA Poppa Bob and Momma Sue) – *For giving Chris a special gift of parental love. Thank you for including us in your family, making us a son and daughter to you.*

Dr. Burton M. Needles, Dr. Michael J. Chehval, Dr. Mary Faller and your staff – *Chris had the best doctors and nurses, because you never gave up hope. May God bless you in your tender loving care for your patients.*

Chris' hospice nurse, Terry Lauck Becker – *You took such loving care of Chris during the hardest part of his race. You will always have a special place in my heart.*

Father Donald Wester – *You helped strengthen our faith during the most trying times of our race and you affirmed our love to keep riding on together.*

Father Christopher Holtmann – *For showing us how to look up to the highest hope of all.*

My Neighbors, "The Cul-de-sac Angels" – *The many times you cut our grass and shoveled snow off our driveway, fixing our garage door, for all the cards, meals, and extra help you've given us, and most especially for your friendship and love. You are the best neighbors.*

My friends at McNair Elementary of the Hazelwood School District – *For your extra support at school and at home so that I could be there for Chris. Go Wildcats!*

Susan Shelton – *For sharing your butterfly with me, which became the first of many while writing this book.*

Christian Bertel – *For reminding me that God's Word will bring me comfort and peace during the darkest days of my grief.*

Trelitha Bryant – *For guiding me to a starting point for the book and your encouragement to ride on with it.*

Toni Saulet – *For helping me fill in some of the blanks of Chris' earlier life which made me admire him even more.*

Karen Schmidt – *For the writing care package you gave me that carried me to the finish line.*

My friends from Armstrong Health and Fitness of Troy, Missouri – *For your support through the 5K Tour de Troy walk/run. Your competitive drive and positive attitude gave Chris a boost to keep going.*

Troop C of the Missouri State Highway Patrol – *Your encouragement and visits with Chris during the hardest time of his race meant so much to him. Thank you for helping me honor his civic duty to our state. May God keep you safe.*

131ˢᵗ Fighter Wing of the Missouri Air National Guard – *For going above and beyond to honor Chris' duty to our country. May God bless you for your service.*

IPMS Chapter of St. Louis and **Mastercon Clubs** – *For sharing your optimism and love of modeling with Chris.*

Momentum Cycles of St. Peters, Missouri – *For sharing your friendship and passion for riding with Chris and for your awesome tribute to him that I'll always remember.*

Jim Heaton at Baue Funeral and Memorial Center of St. Charles, Missouri – *For going above and beyond to help me celebrate and honor Chris' life.*

Rick and Tammy Rooney – *For your beautiful photographic tribute of Chris that I'll always cherish.*

My friends at All Saints Catholic Church and School of St. Peters, Missouri – *I have found a wonderful place of worship to learn more about God's Word and a place to work as a substitute teacher. Your faith and commitment in spreading God's message is an inspiration to me.*

W.G.W. – *While we cried many tears together, we found laughter once again. Ladies, you've been my rock in the hardest place of my life.*

Shelly Michel – *For helping me ride on over those little bumps on the road.*

Laura Schoonover, my hairstylist – *For helping me look beautiful for my author photo shoot.*

My counselor – *For helping me through the most painful time of my life. May God bless your gift in helping others.*

My editor: Cindy O'Hara – *You believed in this story even though my writing needed a lot of work. You've challenged and pushed me beyond what I knew I had in me to become a writer. Thank you for standing by my side to the finish line.*

To you, the reader – *Thank you for picking up this book. I strongly felt the course of my teaching career changed paths to leave after 14 years to write this memoir. It is my hope that you find our story an inspiration to develop a closer relationship with God and ride on victoriously across your finish line with Him.*

There are so many who have touched our lives, and if you do not see your name in this list, please know it is written in my heart.

With love and hugs, Stephanie

Ride On!

Prologue

"You've all been to the stadium and seen the athlete's race. Everyone runs; one wins. Run to win. All good athletes train hard. They do it for the gold medal that tarnishes and fades. But you're after one that's gold eternally."

- 1st Corinthians 9:24 – 25

When you go to a race, you go for the thrill of the competition, to see how someone would win it. After the winner has been declared and the prize has been rewarded, it's over. What do you do then?

You go back to dealing with your reality – *your life* – which is your own personal race. Each of us is in our own kind of race, enjoying the thrills or enduring the different obstacles in it.

What part of the race are you in right now?

Are you on an easy course? One in which your job or career, your finances, your home, and your personal life are all in order. Perhaps you're in the midst of or have already achieved a goal, a dream, experienced joy and love?

Is it a difficult course? Are you in the middle of a war, unemployment, financial problems, or homelessness? Maybe you're dealing with an addiction, an illness, or a disability. Perhaps it's the daily challenge of stress, depression, loneliness, grief.

If you are like me, it's easy to forget to pray when things are going well enough to keep riding on. But pray we must because sometimes you may come to a dead end where things go wrong. You may recognize the road because you've already been on it once, twice, more. You may find yourself struggling on a steep hill, wondering if you'll ever make it to the top and finally reaching the summit and enjoying the thrill of riding downhill, only to crash when you hit a pothole. What will you do then?

I have come to believe that we shouldn't wait for that bike wreck to put on our protective gear. We need to be proactive, because we don't always know what's up ahead or around the corner. But how do we protect ourselves? By believing God's Word.

All great athletes who have won medals have done so with much determination and faith. They *believed* they could win and dug deep within themselves to discover their capacity to achieve their goal. If we deepen our faith, hope, and love, then

"...we are more than conquerors through Jesus who loved us."

- Romans 8:37

Like an athlete, each of us has this amazing will. There is so much more in us than we have ever experienced and it all begins with our faith – our trust in God – to give us the strength we need to keep going in our race. Faith is knowing you can get through the obstacles of your race only with the help of God. Faith is knowing all things are possible with and through Him.

"[We] can do all things through Christ who strengthens [us]."

- Philippians 4:13

Whatever course you are on, keep going – run, ride, walk, or crawl if you have to. Faith is knowing it will all work out, you *will* make it, and victory *will* be yours with Jesus cheering for you at the finish line. It is up to us to grow, to train, to learn, to improve and to perform with endurance our life's race to,

"...press toward the goal for the prize of the upward call in Christ Jesus."

- Philippians 3:14

How did Chris and I persevere in the biggest race of our lives?

Through the long flat stretches, tailwinds, crosswinds, hills, dead ends, blowouts, crashes, and storms, we rode on, side by side across the finish line – victorious.

The Starting Line:
Thursday, September 15th, 2005

"Keep your sight on what is ahead and your eyes directed straight in front of you. Test the ground under your feet and all your ways will be secure. Turn neither to [the] left nor to [the] right and keep your path from evil."

- Proverbs 4:25–27

I was on my lunch break at the elementary school where I taught when I called my fiancé, Chris. I wanted to know how he was feeling after having a biopsy of a lump done the day before. I could barely hear his smooth, strong voice when he answered.

"Chris?"

"Hi babe."

"Did I wake you up?" I started to apologize and he interrupted.

"Steph, I just got off the phone with Dr. Chehval," the urologist who performed the procedure. There was a silence between us that gave me this eerie feeling that something was not right. I couldn't imagine what could be wrong.

"It's cancer."

My knuckles closed around the earpiece tightly as if it could somehow support me. No, I couldn't have heard him correctly.

"I'm sorry, what did you say?"

Chris cleared his throat, "I have cancer."

I looked around the empty staff lounge trying to process the words he had just said to me. Cancer? Chris has cancer? Oh my God. I didn't know what to say.

"Steph?"

"Yes?" I struggled to say the single syllable word.

"Are you okay?"

"Uh-huh," I mumbled and took a deep breath, "How are *you* doing?"

"I'm fine," Chris paused. "Listen Steph, I have to get off the phone. Dr. Chehval recommended an oncologist and I'm waiting to hear from him. I don't want to hang up unless I know for sure that you're alright."

1

"I'm okay," but he wasn't convinced and told me to call him back during my next break later in the afternoon.

"I love you babe. I'll talk to you soon."

"I love you, too," I whispered and stared at the phone, listening to the lifeless tone on the other end of the line. I slowly hung it back on the receiver and tried to make sense of our conversation. How could three words instantly threaten everything wonderful? We just got engaged. And now, Chris has cancer? No. There has to be a mistake. Chris was a healthy man and in excellent physical shape. How could this be possible?

I struggled to breathe. Suddenly feeling desperate, but not sure of what to do, I began pacing around the room when a staff member walked in. We stopped and stared at each other. She took one look at me, quickly turned around and left. I shook my head, sat down at one of the round tables and buried my face in my hands when suddenly the door flew open. I looked up as my fifth grade team and principal rushed into the room.

"Chris has cancer!" I cried out, "Oh my God, Chris has cancer." Sobbing, I collapsed in their comforting arms.

The next thing I knew, my principal arranged for them to drive me to Chris' house.

"Thank you," I whispered.

Amee and Ali put their arm around my shoulders and led me out of the building. I filled them in and they couldn't believe it any more than I could. I slowly climbed in Amee's car feeling completely spent, not wanting to think about it anymore. I sank lower in the passenger seat, closed my eyes and drifted back to when Chris and I met.

It was mid-April 2004 and I was at a party, joking around with one of my friends when a woman I've never seen before joined us. She just stood there, listening to our conversation while keeping her attention on me. I glanced at her from time to time and wondered what was up with her when she interrupted us.

"So, Stephanie, are you married?"

"No," I answered quickly, curious why she wanted to know.

"Are you seeing anyone?"

I shook my head. I was 32 years old and still single.

"I've decided to take a break from dating and explore other things for my life," I told her. I had recently been thinking about adopting a little girl. So much so that I went to a special mass honoring families with adopted children. Since I was adopted, I became so inspired that I started looking into it.

I watched her long, straight blond hair drape over her shoulder as she put her wine glass down on the table. Her 5-foot-6-inch slender frame in a black, short-sleeved dress stood in front of me. The humor was gone from her blue eyes and the soft, sweet tone in her voice changed to an authoritative manner.

"I know you're thinking of doing other things in your life, but I need to tell you something: there *is* someone for you. Don't commit yourself to anything right now. Be patient. God is preparing you for him and He's preparing him for you. When you're ready, you will meet."

Then she smiled that showed off her crimson lips against perfectly white teeth.

"And Stephanie, both of you will meet sooner than you think."

I stared at her, wondering if she was a psychic and how she knew about my faith and belief in God.

She picked up her glass and raised it to me, "Here's to a new beginning!"

I looked at my friend who stood there with wide eyes and her mouth agape.

"Okay," I said slowly, clinking my glass to theirs, "to a new beginning,"

Although I was unaware of this, Chris told me that around the same time, he went for a bike ride with Bob, his best friend, and had dinner with him and his wife, Kelly, one night. These two men shared a strong passion for cycling, family values, protecting their community, and a goofy sense of humor. They were sitting at the kitchen table and my name came up in the conversation. Bob and I knew each other through his grandparents who had been good friends with my parents for many years.

After hearing about me again, Chris leaned forward and challenged Kelly, "Enough talk about this Stephanie. I want to meet her. I'm tired of hearing Stephanie, Stephanie, Stephanie, how great she is and how nice she is. Obviously there is no Stephanie or I would have met her by now. So, bring her on."

Kelly looked over at Bob and then at Chris, "Alright, I'll make a call to ask her and set something up."

"Bring it on. Let's go to the movies, dinner, whatever. It doesn't matter. I'll do anything to meet Stephanie."

3

Several days after their conversation, my phone rang and it was Kelly. I was so surprised to hear from her since it was the first time she had ever called me. I thought maybe she was calling to invite me for a family event, but usually Bob's grandmother would call me about those.

"What's up, Kelly," I asked, puzzled.

"Well, I was wondering if you were seeing anyone."

"No," I answered slowly and she started to tell me about Chris.

"Stephanie, Chris is one of the best people Bob and I know. I think you two have a lot in common and could become friends."

Oh, Kelly is playing Matchmaker. I wasn't sure if I wanted to go through another fix-up. I stared out my kitchen window and watched my dogs, Benji – a white and beige Pomeranian/poodle mix, and Bridget – a black and brown Yorkie, explore the perimeter of the backyard. Something inside of me told me to take a chance.

"Okay. Tell me about him," and I settled in one of the chairs at the table.

"Chris and Bob met in the Highway Patrol and became best friends. Chris now works in the Gaming Division at one of the casinos. He stays in shape by working out, walking his dog, and riding his bike. He's a serious cyclist and competes sometimes. Steph, he is very good looking: he is tall and has black hair, dark brown eyes, and light brown skin."

She wasn't sure about his ethnic background and asked if I was okay about it and I told her that it didn't matter to me.

"So," she paused, "do you think you might be interested in meeting him?"

I stood up and went back to the window. The sun was already peeking behind the trees in preparation for another glorious setting against a clear blue sky. I shook my head, Chris sounded too good to be true. "Kelly, you speak so highly of Chris, but how is it that he is still single?"

"I know, Stephanie. He's such a good man and I want to see him happy with someone. That's when I thought of you and told him about you. He wants to meet you."

"Really? Okay, Kelly, what did you tell Chris?"

She described me as slender and about the same height as her (around 5-feet-4-inches tall), with short brown hair. She described how nice and sweet I was toward others and how close I was to my mother and Bob's grandparents. She told him that I was a teacher who was dedicated to my profession. Just a little bit of this information was enough to intrigue him.

"Stephanie, I'm not trying to put any pressure on you. The two of you seem to share a lot of the same values and both of you are so friendly and a lot of fun which is why I think you'll hit it off. But I want you to be comfortable about this too." Maybe Kelly knew me better than I thought.

I've always felt flattered whenever someone wanted to introduce me to a friend of theirs, but I get so nervous and tongue-tied when I'm put on the spot that I feel lost on what to say or do. The strange thing was I didn't have those feelings this time. Somehow I knew it was going to be okay to meet this particular person.

"Okay, Kelly, tell Chris I'd like to meet him too." She laughed and promised to call soon to set something up.

It took about a month of several phone calls to figure out when all of us could get together. When we thought we could meet one evening, Chris had to work the late shift. We tried another day to meet for brunch, but I had plans with my family. Kelly thought we could play soccer, but it didn't sound like a fun first date to me. I wondered if we were ever going to meet until, finally, we were all free for a movie and dinner at the end of May, which by then was within a week away.

Several days before the date, Kelly called to ask if she could give Chris my number. He wanted to introduce himself and talk with me for a few minutes before we'd meet. I thought it was so considerate of him and told her it was okay. Later on that same day, Chris called. I didn't expect to hear from him so soon.

"Hello. Can I speak with Stephanie?" He spoke in a strong, smooth, sexy tone that made small goose bumps pop up all over my body.

"This is she," I giggled. He laughed and introduced himself then thanked me for letting Kelly give him my number. Throughout the conversation I kept stuttering, but he didn't seem to notice. We talked about how we knew Bob and Kelly. We discovered that we both enjoyed going to the movies and found out our favorite movie series was *Star Wars*. Before hanging up, we agreed to meet in front of the theater a half-an-hour early before Bob and Kelly so we could have a little more time to talk.

"I enjoyed talking with you, Stephanie, and I'm looking forward to meeting you. Until then, with you the force will be, hmmm." Chris said imitating Yoda. Laughing, I told him goodbye and felt a sudden burst of excitement after hanging up the phone. I checked my calendar and realized it was going to be a long three days.

I couldn't stop thinking about the blind date: would we hit it off like Kelly believed or would one of us – or both of us – want to high-tail it out of there? Is he good looking the way Kelly described? Is he really as nice and fun as he seemed on the phone? Will my nerves finally calm down after meeting him or when Bob and Kelly show up? Then I wondered what Chris was doing or if he was thinking about the evening?

Why was I doing this to myself? Kelly said Chris was a great guy so I needed to enjoy the anticipation of meeting him.

By the day of the date, my nerves were so jittery, I took a long, hot shower to help relax and carefully chose white capris and a light, metallic green, sleeveless blouse hoping it would bring out my eyes.

Before I reversed out of my driveway, I gripped the steering wheel and took a deep breath. *Okay, I can do this. Just go with it.*

It didn't take long to get to the theater and I was a few minutes early. I took several more deep breaths to try to calm the fluttering in my stomach. The longer I sat there, the worse I felt and slowly climbed out of the car. I tried to steady my breathing and took my time walking toward the entrance. I was about 30 feet away when I saw Chris come out of one of the doors in a light gold T-shirt with navy shorts and sandals. We spotted each other right away and when he smiled at me, all of the butterflies suddenly calmed down. I knew he was the one I was supposed to meet.

Chris would tell you that after he saw me, he thought, "Yep, Bob was right. She is cute."

When I got closer, Chris took off his sunglasses and walked a couple of long strides to meet me and shook my hand. I looked down and couldn't tell whose hand was whose. We seemed to bond together. Chris didn't miss a beat and eased us into a conversation, making me laugh. I don't remember what we talked about because I couldn't help noticing how his chocolate-colored eyes were focused on me. I wondered if I had finally met my tall, dark, and handsome man of my dreams.

Chris told me later that he felt an immediate connection with me and was so excited about it that he hoped I felt the same way.

It seemed only a few minutes passed instead of a half-an-hour when Chris pointed out that Bob and Kelly just drove into the parking lot. He asked if I would be willing to play a joke on them with humor in his eyes that made him look like an excited little boy.

"Okay, what do you want to do?"

"Great," he said. I didn't think he could smile any bigger. "What we'll do is stand closer together and lean into each other's necks to give the illusion that we are kissing like the actors did in those old black and white movies."

"Wait a minute," I stepped back and tilted my head, "What?"

Chris laughed and put his hands up, "I promise it's all in good fun and I will be a perfect gentleman. But if you don't feel comfortable to do this, I understand. I just want to get Kelly."

I closely scrutinized him and thought about what he had said.

I nodded slowly and pointed my finger at him, "But no monkey business."

"If I tell you each move I make, will that be easier for you?" I giggled and stepped closer to him. I couldn't believe I was actually going through with this.

"First, I'll put my hands on your back and if you'd like, you can put your hands on my shoulders." Chris asked if I was doing okay so far and once I looked into his eyes, I was lost and nodded.

He suggested leaning in closer while promising he wouldn't try anything funny. We kept laughing and I doubted we looked convincing at all. Chris whispered they were close and we broke apart. Bob and Kelly slowly walked toward us with their mouths wide open. I glanced at Chris who was smiling. *There was no way we were believable.*

"Uh, what's up buddy?" Bob asked slowly, shaking Chris' hand.

"Nothing much," Chris answered.

"It's not what you think," I whispered when we hugged. But they still held that shock-and-awe expression. To keep things going, Chris told them that the movie was about to start and Bob went to buy tickets while Kelly kept eyeing the both of us. She gave short answers when Chris asked about their three kids. I wondered what I had gotten myself into and when I looked up at him, he winked at me. *Oh boy. Why did he have to be so cute?*

Throughout the movie, Kelly kept glancing over at us, then whispered in Bob's ear and he'd hush her. *Really? I couldn't believe we were that convincing.* I told myself that I'd have to have a little chat with Chris. I didn't want our friends to get the wrong impression.

After the movie, we carpooled together to a nearby restaurant for dinner. Without realizing it, I think Bob played one up on Chris when he turned on the song, *Dancing Queen* by Abba and told me it was Chris' favorite song. I questioned Chris, but he shook his head, laughing. I joined Bob and Kelly singing it to him while he kept trying to poke some jibes back at Bob.

At the restaurant, Chris kept up the joke by putting his arm around the back of my chair and giving me a few long glances. I thought it was enough and tried to glare at him, but he smiled and winked at me and I'd melt all over again.

Before I knew it, it was the end of the date and Chris was walking me to my car. I noticed he wasn't as talkative and slowed down his pace a bit. After I unlocked my door, I turned around to say goodbye. He looked down at the ground and then at me.

"Would you like to go out on another date?"

I paused, studying him. He held a hopeful expression that was so adorable.

"Yes," I answered. "I'd like to see you again." He smiled and opened my door and before he closed it, he bent down until we were face-to-face. This time, he paused. I held my breath and wondered if he was going to kiss me.

"Drive home safely," he said, smiling, and closed the door. I waved goodbye and laughed to myself.

I wasn't home 15 minutes when my phone rang. Chris wanted to make sure I made it home okay and to let me know that he had a good time. He thanked me for being a good sport about the joke and thought we pulled it off, laughing at Bob's and Kelly's reaction. He promised me that he would tell them when the time was right.

After we said goodnight, I thought of how nice it was for him to call. This told me that I was on his mind, just as he was on mine. And I was thrilled.

Together for a Reason

"I believe God brought us together for a reason. I believe the day we met, our lives were being blessed."

- Author Unknown

"Steph," said Amee, bringing me back, "we're almost at Chris' house." I looked out the window and recognized the houses in the subdivision. I pulled down the visor and shook my head at my reflection, it would be impossible to look okay. I straightened my hair then dug into my purse in search for something that would provide me with a miraculous makeover within the next few minutes. All I had was powder and lipstick. It was better than nothing.

Amee slowly drove up the driveway to a three-bedroom ranch with soft gray siding and red brick. The beige truck and the shiny black SUV were still parked in the garage, facing us, as Amee put the gear into Park and Ali carefully drove my car next to us. I sat there, clutching my purse.

"What do I say to him, Amee?" She looked at the house and then at me.

"Just be there for him, Steph, and that alone will be enough."

I took a deep breath and got out of the car. Ali was already by my side, pressing the keys in my hand.

"Steph, I know everything is going to work out. You and Chris will get married and have a family that you've always dreamed of."

"Ali is right. Stay strong and believe. We're here for you," Amee said and the three of us hugged.

"Thank you for getting me here," I whispered.

I let go of my friends, spun around, raced through the garage in between the cars, and flew through the door.

"Chris?" I shouted.

He was walking up the steps from the basement and I froze. Neither of us said anything. I couldn't read his expression and wondered what he was thinking. When he reached the top step, Chris reached out to me. I dropped my things and grabbed him. I tried so hard to be strong but the tears took over. Chris wrapped his arms tightly around me. When we finally pulled apart, he tilted my chin and kissed me.

"I knew you'd come," he whispered.

He wiped the tears from my cheeks then led me into the living room and we sat down on the couch. Chris rubbed his forehead and took several deep breaths.

"When Dr. Chehval told me that it was cancer, I felt this fear unlike anything I've ever felt before," he sighed, "but after hanging up the phone, I wasn't afraid anymore. Steph, I'm pissed! Shit. Cancer?" and he punched the armrest.

Speechless, I held his hand.

"You know what, Steph? Whatever this is, it's messing with the wrong body. I'm going to beat it."

Somehow I found my voice.

"Chris, I believe you and if anyone can beat cancer, you can."

He squeezed my hand and smiled sweetly, "Thanks, babe. I'm glad you're here. You showed me that I'm not alone in this and I have you by my side. I can see how much you love me and I'm deeply touched. I'm a lucky man. I love you so much."

I lost whatever strength I had left and burst into tears again.

"I love you, too. But I'm the one who is lucky and there is no one I want to be with more than you," I said. He leaned over and kissed me again. I laid my head on his shoulder and sat with him for a long time.

Suddenly the phone rang, disturbing the silence of our thoughts and we jumped. Chris raced into the kitchen to answer it.

"This is Christopher," I heard him say and I knew it had to be the oncologist he had been waiting to hear from. I walked over to his side and watched him write down the information he was given, nodding, "Yes, I can make that appointment. Thank you." He hung up the phone and smiled, "Okay, we're all set."

I looked at what he wrote: *"Dr. Needles, Monday, September 19th, 4 p.m."*

I raised my eyebrows, "Uh, your doctor's name is Needles?" He glanced at the paper and we started to laugh. It was perfect.

"Well, I guess with a last name like that, why not become a doctor. Besides, he's supposed to be one of the best."

"Let's hope he is, Chris."

Chris wanted to get out of the house for a while and decided he was in the mood for a turtle sundae from Fritz's Frozen Custard, a local ice cream parlor, and a strawberry/banana sundae sounded good to me. Sometimes, having ice cream is just the right ingredient to cheer up a soul, even for a short while.

After we got back, we took his dog, D'Artagnon, a 90 pound black, white, and gray Alaskan Malamute, for a short walk. This little bit of exercise was enough to take some of the edge off of us. Chris admitted that he was feeling anxious about getting through the weekend before the meeting with Dr. Needles, but was glad that it was sooner rather than later. We brainstormed about how we could get through the next three days. I had teacher meetings all day on Friday and Chris was scheduled to work the three-to-eleven shifts all weekend. We planned to meet for dinner during his break Friday night. We thought that working in our yards on Saturday morning would help relieve some of the stress and he'd go to work while I'd see a movie with a girlfriend. Then we'd attend Sunday morning church service and go out for brunch before his shift. By having a plan to stay busy, we hoped the appointment would be here before we knew it.

It was beginning to get dark and I knew I had to get home to take care of Benji and Bridget. We were still processing everything and it was too much for one person to handle alone. I kept making excuses not to leave. I slowly searched for the car keys in my purse and kept stalling.

"How about I come over and stay overnight with you after I get D'Artagnon settled?"

"Are you sure?" I asked, shocked. He smiled sweetly, kissed me, and promised to be over soon. I realized he needed to be with me as much as I needed him.

After Chris arrived, we suddenly felt drained and worn out from the day. We tried to watch a movie, but neither of us could keep our eyes open and decided to turn in early. Chris was already comfortable in my bed when I carefully climbed in next to him. He looked so peaceful and I guessed he was already asleep. I put my hand on his chest and could feel his strong heartbeat. He smiled a little and rested his hand over mine. I cuddled closer to him and rested my head on his shoulder. I looked at his strong, healthy body and couldn't imagine there was a cancerous tumor inside of him. What kind of cancer was it? What kind of treatment would he have to endure to fight it? How would it affect his cycling and walking D'Artagnon, his job at the casino and at the Air National Guard, doing chores in the house and in the yard, working on his military models? How would this affect us? *I don't want to lose him!* I couldn't imagine my life without him. *Oh God, could this just be a bad dream?* I shut my eyes and hoped that my clock radio would wake me up. But I knew better and the tears started again. Chris stirred, tightened his arms around me and kissed my forehead.

"It's going to be okay, Steph. We're together and that's the most important thing right now. Just focus on us," he whispered. I snuggled in his arms and I found myself back to the moment when we realized we were falling in love.

It was an unusually cool day for August in 2004 when Chris and I decided to spend the afternoon at a park near my house. We strolled around the lake, enjoying the sights around us. We laughed at a family of ducks scrambling and competing over pieces of dried bread that a little girl and her mother threw at them. We admired the patience of a grandpa teaching his young grandson how to throw a fishing line into the water. And we listened to a small group of 4-or-5-year-olds playing on the playground while their mothers sat on a bench close by. There was no need to talk. We stole a glance at each other as if we already knew what the other was thinking. It was so surreal to experience this kind of closeness after dating two months.

Chris led me to a gazebo that was set apart from the lake and asked me to sit with him, draping his arm over my shoulders and held my hand. I looked down and wondered again, which hand was his and which was mine. We seemed to fit together in the same way a puzzle piece connects perfectly with all the other pieces around it, completing the picture. I was about to tell him this until I gazed into his adoring brown eyes and forgot what I was going to say. He leaned in and kissed me deeply. Maybe it was the soft breeze, or maybe it was the magic within the park, or maybe it was that unexpected, amazing moment that was the right time for us, but this kiss was unlike any other we had shared. It felt as if we had come together as one.

When we broke apart, Chris whispered sweetly in my ear, "Thank you," and held me close for a long time.

My stomach fluttered excitedly and I felt like I was floating even though I knew I was sitting on a wooden bench next to him. I winked at him then blew him a kiss and sang, "We go together, like a wink and a smile!"

"Funny girl," he laughed. He stood up, pulled me close to him and kissed me again.

Several days later, Chris walked me to my door at the end of our date and I noticed he looked uncomfortable as if he didn't know what to do next. He quickly kissed me good night and spun on his heels. I wondered what had gotten into him and watched him get into his truck. I started to put my key in the doorknob and the next thing I knew, I was swept around. Just as I got ready to scream, Chris kissed me again. Holding my hands, he said,

"Stephanie, I've enjoyed all the times we've spent together this summer. I love looking into your eyes and seeing you smile. I hope to make you smile more. What I'm trying to say is, Steph – I love you." He spoke so fast that I didn't catch on right away.

"Oh, okay," I said and gave him a hug. He stood there for a moment, nodded, and then walked briskly back to his truck and drove off.

After I got into the house, I leaned against my door, "Wait a minute." I bumped my head and realized that Chris just told me he loved me. *And what did I do? I sent him away.* I felt like such an idiot.

I slowly walked into my bedroom and sat on my bed. I thought about our kiss in the gazebo and whispered in the empty room, "That was the moment when I fell in love with you, Chris." I wondered what was going through his mind. *Have I blown it?*

There was so much I needed to tell him. The only way I knew I could get it all out was to write him a letter and give it to him the next time I saw him – that is if there would be a next time.

"Chris, the moment I saw you, I knew you were the man I was supposed to meet. You've become my unexpected and my life took a turn for the better. I thought I was happy before I met you but I've experienced what true happiness is by the special man you are: your adoring eyes, your laugh, the sincere way you speak, and the kindness you showed me all became a part of my life. I have never seen so much gentleness in one person. Without knowing it, you were slowly making a place in my heart and as you unfolded yourself to me, I discovered the man of my dreams.

I realize now that I had never known what it meant to be in love until you shared those three lovely words to me under a night full of stars with endless possibilities.

Now I am telling you in the bright sunlight full of hope and dreams: Chris, I love you too."

After I reread the letter, I knew it was perfect. I just hoped I didn't mess things up between us before having the chance to give it to him.

The next day, I called Chris early in the morning. He sounded so happy to hear from me and we made plans to go to Bob's grandfather's birthday party.

When we showed up at Bob's grandparents' place, he stepped in and proudly introduced his best friend to his family. Chris fit in easily, talking and joking with everyone. He took the time to talk with Grandpa and shared some Navy stories and then complimented Grandma on the pretty flowers in her yard. I felt deeply touched by the kindness and sincerity he showed them. How did I get so lucky with this man? After lunch, I took Chris on a tour around the neighborhood and brought him to the lake where Grandpa and my father taught me how to swim when I was a little girl. It was one of my favorite places and I knew this was where I wanted to give Chris my letter.

"I have something for you," I whispered. I took a deep breath, reached into my pocket for the letter and gave it to him. I stood there in front of him on the small sandy beach while he read it. Slowly and carefully, he folded the letter. Not sure of what to do next, I dug my hands into my pockets and kicked a rock I found on the ground. He wrapped his hands around my waist and pulled me close. I looked into his eyes.

"Yes, Chris, I love you," I whispered.

"I'm so happy, Steph," he laughed. "I thought maybe I rushed too quickly or, worse, that I blew it. But I don't have to worry anymore. That day in the gazebo is constantly playing in my mind. That kiss, Steph, was the moment I fell in love with you. You have become 'my unexpected' too. A lasting and loving relationship is not built within a few months. It's built over a lifetime of care and nurturing. We can't learn all there is to know about each other in a few months or a year. That learning is a constant process that can take a lifetime. It's what makes a relationship stronger and the love for each other more powerful. It all takes commitment and effort. I am committed to you, Stephanie and I'm sincerely in love with you. You're always in my thoughts and my heart smiles every time I think of you. We have so much to look forward to and experience together, and I am prepared for a lifetime of learning and growing with you. My heart is yours." Then he kissed me.

Treasuring the memory of that moment, I laid there next to my fiancé and felt his arms loosen its grip. I opened my eyes to check on Chris and he was already sleeping soundly. I kissed his cheek gently so I wouldn't startle him and followed his breathing until my body finally relaxed. Just before I dozed off, I thanked God for bringing this special man into my life and prayed for His protection and healing over him.

Moments

"We do not remember days, we remember moments."

- Author Unknown

I woke up and saw I was alone. I wondered if it was just a bad dream after all. My body felt heavy as I struggled to get out of bed. I slowly made my way into the kitchen and jumped when Chris and my dogs came in through the back door.

"Are you okay? What happened?"

I leaned against the counter and Chris was already by my side, "It was a bad dream, wasn't it?" He held me close.

"I know, Steph. I hoped so too when I woke up. Then I saw you and I knew." I hugged him tightly, not wanting to let him go. "But you know what, we'll always have each other no matter what and we need to keep going together side by side, like how we ride our bikes." I smiled and thought of the time when we first rode together.

During the spring of 2005, Chris' enthusiasm about riding inspired me to ride a bike again. He was like a kid in a toy store at the cycle shop, checking out so many bikes. There was a lot more to a bicycle than I realized as I listened in on the conversations between him and the salespeople. I didn't understand a lot of the lingo, so I focused on the style and color I wanted, but Chris had certain standards of what kind of bike I should get: a hybrid bicycle – so I could ride on the road and on the trail – with an aluminum frame, straight handlebars and clip pedals. He also found the right helmet, gloves, shoes, and clothes for me. I understood the need for a helmet and the special shoes but I thought the shorts with padding on the bottom were a bit overboard.

"Seriously, Chris, do I really need these?" shaking the shorts at him.

"I promise that after the first ride, you won't ever ride a bike without them," Chris said, laughing.

Chris set up my bike on a stand at my house so I could practice clicking my shoes in and out of the pedals. After about a week, I felt ready to ride and we went out to a park near his house. Chris showed me how he clicked his shoe in the pedal, then started pedaling and clicked in the other foot in one smooth, graceful movement. Watching him closely, I thought it was simple enough to do.

I straddled my bike, clicked my right foot in and then started pedaling, but my left foot was stranded. I couldn't figure out how to get it in the pedal and ride at the same time. I tried to see what I was doing, but I started to lose control of the bike and panicked. I suddenly felt a fear of crashing. I held my breath and tightened my grip on the handlebars as if it would prevent me from falling over. I stepped on the pedal and pushed it to keep the bike moving. After many futile attempts, my foot finally clicked into place during the third lap around the parking lot. I took a deep breath to calm down. *Maybe I should have a sign on my back similar to the ones for new drivers on the road, only mine would read, "New cyclist, stay far away!"*

"You did it Steph. The more you practice, the better you'll get at it. Now let's ride." Chris' enthusiasm was contagious and I started to relax. He rode next to me and began to teach me about my bicycle and how to change the gears.

When we were getting thirsty, Chris showed me how to get the water bottle while riding. He lowered himself slightly, pulled out the bottle from its holder, took a quick drink and put it back in one swift motion. *Could there be a ballet on cycling?*

The first time I tried to get it, my bike wobbled and I straightened up quickly.

"Never mind, I'm not really thirsty," even though my mouth felt drier than toast.

"You can do it, Steph. Try again."

I picked up my pace then reached down, gripped the bottle with my right hand and yanked it out of its holder. I struggled to steady my bike while drinking as much as I could. I bent down to put it back, but kept missing the holder. Seeing I was slowing down, I picked up my speed and tried again, but dropped it and the bottle rolled off to the side of the trail. Chris told me to keep riding, went to get it for me, and then handed it back to me. I shook my head.

"You have to have your water, try again." I took a deep breath and was able to put the bottle back in its place. "There you go. Let's keep riding."

Chris kept teaching me about my bike and I started to feel more at ease until I saw a steep hill ahead of us.

"Uh, Chris, we're not going up that hill, are we?"

17

"What do you mean? Hills are your friends. Just follow my cues when to shift your gears. Come on, you can do it." Feeling like I had no choice, I obeyed Chris' commands and discovered that the pedals weren't so hard to push, but keeping the pace up the hill was arduous. I leaned forward and imagined I was Thomas the Little Engine that Could, repeating to myself, *I think I can, I think I can, I think I can.* I was within several feet from the top when suddenly my feet began to spin out of control. Somehow, my chain got loose. I don't know how I did it, but I unclipped my left foot from the pedal and stopped. I knew I had to be pushing Chris' patience at this point. He smiled when he got off his bike and easily snapped the chain back in its place. He put my gear where it should be and showed me which one to be in while riding up the hill. We got back on our bikes and I was able to click my shoe back in the pedal on the first try.

"That's my girl."

I laughed and we rode the rest of the way back to our starting point without any more problems. I was starting to feel confident until we came to another steep hill, only this time it was on a curvy path. Chris reminded me how to shift the gears one at a time and I slowly climbed the hill. When I reached the top, I started to celebrate until I saw a long slope ahead of me. *Oh come on!*

Chris encouraged me, telling me I could do it, so I put my head down close to the handlebars and pressed forward. I didn't stop pedaling until I finally reached the flat surface at the top of the hill.

"You did it, Steph." I gasped for air while we circled the parking lot and watched Chris unclip his shoe and stop his bike. *Okay, I already did this once, I can do it again.* But my legs felt like jello and my lower backside was throbbing. I slowed down to free my right foot and the next thing I knew I was leaning to the left. I was sure I looked just like a tree being cut down falling over to the side and I could have sworn I heard someone yell out, *Timber!* Well, that was me on my brand new bike. But Chris made it in the nick of time, catching me just before my shoulder hit the ground and pulled me up.

"That was close. Are you okay?"

"I'm fine." I snapped. Chris raised his eyebrows and walked away. I know I should have been relieved but I was so frustrated that I didn't get out of the pedals on my own and it was so humiliating to fall down with my bike. I nursed the road rash on my left leg and calmed down.

"I'm sorry. I was really embarrassed, but you were quick to my rescue. Thanks."

Chris pulled down his sunglasses enough for me to see the humor in his eyes, "It was my pleasure, baby," he said in a deep voice.

Reminiscing about our first bike ride, we laughed while we were eating breakfast and it really cheered us up. Chris washed up the dishes for me so I could finish getting ready for a full day of meetings. When it was time to leave, I followed Chris' truck out of my subdivision and waved goodbye to him.

After I parked my car in the school lot, another wave of tears flooded from my eyes. Gripping the steering wheel, I prayed.

Oh God, I don't know how to handle this. I'm so angry and sad this has happened to Chris. I need to be strong for him and I can't do this without You.

I don't know how long I sat there but I knew I had to get going. I quickly walked into the main entrance of the quiet building, hoping to make it upstairs to my classroom without seeing anyone. But several of my colleagues saw me and rushed over to offer support. I couldn't find my voice to speak. All I could do was nod as the tears came again.

At the announcement that the workshop was about to begin, I had a chance to run to my classroom for some solitude. I dropped into my chair and laid my head down on my desk.

Oh God, I feel so weak. I can't do this without you. Please help me. Thank you for the loving care of my friends here.

After a few minutes of deep breathing, I calmed down, grabbed my notepad and pen and headed back downstairs.

The meeting had already started so I snuck in the back of the room quietly and sat in the chair between Amee and Ali. I tried to focus but my mind kept wandering. I didn't realize how bad I was doing until Ali pressed a note into my hand. *Don't worry*, it read. *I'm taking notes for you to look at later. We're all here for you, Steph.*

"Thank you," I whispered and more tears threatened. I took several deep breaths to keep them in control. I tried to listen to the speaker but couldn't stop thinking about Chris. *Cancer.* I shivered and felt the goose bumps dotting my arms and legs. I was afraid – deep within my core. I wondered if this was the kind of fear Chris told me about. Suddenly I realized he was all alone while I had caring people around me. He needed someone there for him too. He needed Bob. The first chance I had, I rushed back to my classroom, grabbed my cell phone from my purse, and ran downstairs and out the front doors. I welcomed the fresh, cool breeze on my face and paced back and forth on the sidewalk, waiting for Kelly to answer. The phone rang on and on.

"Oh, please be there," I whispered and started to think of what to say in case I had to leave a message, when Kelly finally answered,

"Hey Stephanie, I'm sorry I couldn't get to the phone right away…"

"Kelly, where's Bob?" I interrupted.

"Bob is at work right now. What's up?" Hoping I was doing the right thing, I stuttered over my words.

"I had this strong feeling to call you. Can you find Bob? Chris needs his best friend right now."

"I can find him, but what's going on?"

"Kelly, I don't know how to say this or the right way to say it," I paused, struggling to say the words again out loud. "Chris has cancer."

There was a long silence between us. I leaned against the red brick building. I didn't know what else to say.

"Stephanie, did you just say, 'Chris has cancer'?" Kelly stammered.

"Yes," I answered weakly and told her about the diagnosis. The shock in her voice was instantly gone.

"Chris is a very strong man. He is going to pull through this. He needs you to be there for him, Stephanie. You need to be strong with him."

I was amazed at the determination in her voice and felt some of her strength. She promised to call Bob right away and have him get a hold of Chris.

I don't know how I got through the rest of the day, but by the grace of God I felt some of that strength I prayed for earlier and was able to stay focused on my work. By the end of the day, I was drained and was anxious to get home. As I walked out of the building, I found one of my dearest friends standing by her car in the parking lot. She was one of the substitute teachers I worked with and we had grown close over the years and I nicknamed her "Teddie Momma." I burst into tears all over again and ran into her outstretched arms.

"Oh, baby girl," she whispered and prayed over me. She slipped a scripture from Joshua 1:9 in my hand and quoted it.

"It is I who command you; be strong, then, and be valiant. Do not tremble or be afraid, because Yahweh, your God, is with you wherever you go."

I stayed in the comfort of her loving arms and thought about those words. I was overwhelmed by the support and kindness from everyone. It was as if God worked through them to carry me for awhile. I hugged Teddie and thanked her for being there for me. I couldn't wait to share the scripture with Chris later when we would meet for dinner.

I stood by the water fountain at the main entrance of the casino and found myself mesmerized by the different directions the water sprayed, how they would cross each other, low then high, in a rhythmic fashion. After another round of it, I turned and found Chris a short distance away walking toward me. I was almost breathless. The man knew how to look good in a suit. He kept checking the activity around him while stealing a glance at me several times. I stood there in awe as he casually placed his hand on my back and leaned over for a quick kiss.

"Hi babe, you look nice. Have you been waiting long?"

I shook my head and fanned myself.

Chris tilted his head, "Are you hot?" he asked.

"Oh yes, and so are you, strutting in a cool cat kind of way – very suave and sexy."

"Funny girl," Chris laughed. "Come on, let's go and get something to eat before you fall in this fountain. I'm starving."

We seemed to pick up where we left off and things felt as normal between us as much as it had before the diagnosis. I told Chris about my day, sharing my amazement at God's love and how He takes care of us through others when we need Him the most. Chris agreed and told me that Bob called him.

"Somehow, I just knew you needed him, Chris." I confided that I got a hold of Kelly to find Bob and he looked at me surprised.

"You were right, I did need my best friend and he was there for me."

I told him about Teddie waiting for me in the school parking lot and then I showed him the scripture. His eyes got big and he smiled.

"I'm not afraid," Chris said, sitting back in his chair and fingered the scripture. "I'll be strong and I'm going to beat this thing."

"With God's help, we can beat this together."

I couldn't stop admiring my tall, dark, and handsome fiancé in his charcoal suit and wondered how I would handle seeing him in a tuxedo on our wedding day.

"What are you thinking about?" Chris asked, interrupting my thoughts and I told him.

He became very quiet, took my left hand, scrunched his eyebrows together, and studied my engagement ring."

"Do you still want to marry me?" he asked.

I gazed into those brown eyes that I adored so much and thought about two incredible moments earlier that summer.

We had been together for a year and we decided to celebrate by going on our first vacation together to Oahu, Hawaii. We had to go to Pearl Harbor before we did anything else on the island. As a veteran of the United States Navy, Chris wanted to pay his respects to the fallen sailors laid to rest there. We arrived early and there was already a long line of people waiting to get inside. After buying our tickets for a film presentation and the ferry to the U.S.S. Arizona, we had plenty of time to explore the museum. There were newspaper clippings, black and white photos, videos of news reports, preserved artifacts, and dioramas of the ships and of Japan's attack. Chris didn't want to miss a thing, perusing every detail and taking pictures.

The auditorium was packed as people watched the documentary of President Roosevelt declaring war on Japan and clips of the attack. Afterwards, it was so quiet it felt as if you could almost hear the whispers of the fallen.

Chris, I noticed, stood prouder and walked with an air of confidence and strength. There were many different nationalities around us and despite our differences in where we came from, in the language we spoke, or the religion we practiced, we all shared the same feelings of sadness and awe, respect and honor for the sailors at rest there.

We stood together on the bridge overlooking the tomb of the magnificent ship, and then one by one, pink and white plumerias, bright yellow and red hibiscus, and colorful leis dotted the silver water. You could see tiny bubbles of oil that were still leaking from the depths of the ship popping sporadically at the surface. Chris kept his arm around my waist and held me close to him. None of us could imagine the agony of that fateful day, but America had grown stronger and we could feel it in our hearts standing there. The only sound that could be heard were the cameras clicking and the soft breeze flapping the American flag directly above us.

After we exited off the ferry, Chris wasn't next to me. I looked around and found him off to the side, facing the U.S.S. Arizona Memorial. I watched him take off his sunglasses and wipe his eyes. Then he pushed his shoulders back, held his head high, and saluted. He put his sunglasses on, turned around, made his way toward me, and we left in silence.

We were coming to the end of our vacation with a couple of days left and I was beginning to wonder if Chris would propose to me. We knew we were right for each other and we talked about marriage and having a family. I thought maybe Chris would ask me to marry him here of all places. The question that kept repeating in my mind was, would he? All I could do was hope.

Chris made a reservation for a sunset luau so we could fully appreciate the experience. At the beginning of the festivities, we stood on the smooth sandy beach and watched two fishermen cast their nets into the calm ocean, demonstrating a Hukilau, the Hawaiian way of fishing. The setting was as surreal as the sweet perfumed fragrances from the tropical flowers mixed with the salty ocean breeze. The sun began to drop into the horizon, painting the sky in hues of orange, purple, and blue, cooling the warm air.

"Going, going, going, gone," Chris whispered and the sun disappeared.

I turned around and circled my hands around his neck. Chris followed my gaze and saw the stars already dotting against the dark blue sky. He tilted my chin and kissed me. It was such a magical moment, I wondered if he would propose. But the spell was broken by someone blowing into a conch shell, announcing that the luau dinner was about to begin.

Afterwards, Chris suggested taking a walk on the beach. By this time, the night sky was twinkling with a million stars and more waves brushed gently against the shore. Chris was talking but I was so mesmerized by the tropical beauty around us that I hardly heard what he was saying. Suddenly he stopped and knelt down on one knee in front of me and held both of my hands.

"Steph, when we met, I had no idea how much my life was going to change. I discovered what love truly is with you. You've become my best friend and the love of my life. I can't think of anything that would make me happier than to spend the rest of my life with you. I promise to make you happy, love you, and take care of you for the rest of yours. Will you marry...?"

"Yes!" I screamed. He laughed and swept me into his arms.

"Thank you," he whispered in my ear and kissed me.

Chris squeezed my hand, bringing me back to the present. I looked around the restaurant to regroup. He was studying me, still waiting for my answer. I let go, reached over to his left hand and held it in mine. I looked into his eyes and felt such a deep love for him and from him.

"I do," I said confidently.

He brought my hand to his lips with that sweet smile that made my knees quiver, "I can't wait."

On Your Mark

"Keep sight on what is ahead and your eyes directed straight in front of you."

- Proverbs 4:25

Even though the weekend flew by, Monday seemed to take its time. When the final dismissal bell rang and the last of my students excitedly left the classroom, I snatched my purse from the desk drawer and bolted out of my chair. The last thing I did before racing out of the room was slam the light switch down, causing dark shadows to play across the ceiling, the desks, the walls, and on the floor. The lack of light and the shadows made me uneasy, almost as if they portrayed Chris' outcome. I shivered. I flipped the light back on and took a deep breath. *Oh God, shine your light of wisdom and show us what to do.* I closed my eyes and let my hand drop over the switch, turning my back against the darkness.

I darted around the slow-paced cars hoping to get to the cancer center within 20 minutes before the appointment. It was easy to find the small brick building and I saw Chris walking with his oldest brother, Mark, and his wife, Toni, across the barren parking lot. They drove in from Kansas to be there for him. I ran to the entrance and Chris squeezed my hand.

"Hi babe. We have plenty of time," he whispered. When we stepped through the automatic doors, I was surprised at how bright it was in the wide open room. *Thank you, God, for the light in this place.*

Throughout the lobby, chairs and loveseats in soft cream with a hint of mauve and blue hues were conveniently and purposefully scattered, accompanied by mahogany tables with various informational brochures and current newspapers and magazines. When we turned toward the elevators, there was soft, calming music from the piano playing itself off to the side of the entrance. Chris ran his finger down the list of doctors from a plaque on the wall and found Dr. Needles' office. We exited the elevator and the view of the lobby added to the serenity of the place. We walked to the end of the hall through the large double doors into a spacious waiting room decorated in deep colors of hunter green, navy, and maroon that enhanced the quietness of the place.

We were the only ones there and I wondered if we were the last appointment of the day. Chris signed in on the clipboard and the receptionist told him to fill out the new patient paperwork while she copied his insurance card. Several minutes later, a nurse stepped out from the closed door and called Chris' name. He handed over the paperwork to her as she led us into a long, narrow room where they would check his weight, temperature, and blood pressure before seeing the doctor. Stunned, I watched her work with Chris. *What? How often would he have to come here?*

But it didn't faze him. Chris let the nurse take his vitals and pretended to leap off the scale.

After recording the information in his crisp new medical file (that I would soon come to hate), we were led down a long hallway, past many rooms, until she opened the door of one and told us that Dr. Needles would be with us shortly. Chris sat on the examining table and we settled into the hard chairs. I opened my notebook to the page of questions Chris wanted to ask. Looking over them, my heart was pounding so hard I was sure it echoed in the tiny room. I caught Chris' eye and he smiled. I started to calm down when the door swung open and an averaged-height man with salt and pepper hair, dark rimmed glasses, and wearing a white lab coat entered. He shook Chris' hand first, and then greeted the rest of us. He sat down on the small stool and asked a series of questions to learn more about Chris' medical background. Overall, Chris was a very healthy 46-year-old man who never smoked and had only a few drinks in his life. The only history of cancer in his family was from his mother who died of breast cancer after it recurred the second time. No one else had been diagnosed with cancer. Dr. Needles wanted to examine Chris so we stepped out of the room. I stood next to a stained-glassed window in the hallway and rested my head on it, allowing the primary colors to dance on my face. *Lord, I have to believe that we're in the right place with the right doctor. Show us how we can fight this cancer.*

The door jerked open and Chris waved for us to come back in.

Dr .Needles finished writing his notes then crossed his arms across his chest and sighed.

This can't be good.

"The mass located inside the urethra is called 'urethral cancer.'" He paused.

"I've never heard of it," Chris said, puzzled.

"This is a rare type of cancer in which malignant cells form in the tissues of the urethra," Dr. Needles explained. "I've already called the cancer centers in Houston, Chicago, and New York to get input on how to treat it." Focusing on Chris, he continued, "Because this cancer is so rare, there is no consensus on what to do to cure it – chemotherapy, radiation, surgery, or a combination of any of these three."

I froze. I couldn't bring myself to write what I had just heard and kept staring at my notebook, afraid to see Chris' reaction. A heavy weight filled my chest and my heart sped up. *Chris has a rare cancer. The doctors cannot agree on how to treat it?*

All at once, Chris, Mark, and Toni began firing questions at the doctor:

"What is the cause of this cancer?"

"How big is the tumor?"

"What stage is it in?"

"Is this the only tumor?"

"Will Chris have to do chemo and radiation to treat it?"

"Can it be removed surgically and then do treatment?"

Dr. Needles waited patiently, listening to them while I struggled to keep up the notes.

"We need to do some tests to learn more about the cancer and hopefully we'll find some answers. I recommend a complete blood count, an MRI of the pelvic area, a CT-scan of the lungs, liver, and abdomen, and a PET scan of Chris' body."

We sat there in silence. I wrote the long list, feeling overwhelmed. Finally, I looked at Chris, who was rubbing his chin thoughtfully.

"Okay, let's do it," he said. Dr. Needles wrote out the orders and explained that we may or may not be able to do the PET scan – it depended on the type of health insurance Chris had. I stopped writing and spoke for the first time.

"Really? Do we have to worry about insurance coverage on top of this?" *God, can you take care of this? This is too much already!*

No one answered me.

"I don't know," said Dr. Needles, "but talk to Nancy who deals with insurance companies. She can work wonders for our patients."

"How soon can I get in for these tests?" asked Chris.

Dr. Needles explained that one of the receptionists would put the order in and Chris would get a phone call with the time, place, and instructions. He reassured all of us that he would continue researching for a treatment regimen and he hoped to have some ideas after reviewing the test results.

"When we meet again, we'll go over everything and decide what to do," said Dr. Needles.

It felt as if we had just gotten on a rollercoaster and took a sudden drop and turn after a long climb. With the orders in his hands, we quickly followed Chris, who was already halfway down the hall toward the receptionist. We found out there was a lab on the second floor for the blood work where he could go without an appointment. She told us that Chris would be able to get in for the other tests before returning to Dr. Needles. Checking my calendar, I saw that we'd have to wait 10 days to find out more about this cancer. *How are we going to get through this long waiting period?*

While Chris went to the lab, I walked around the small library on the main floor, searching for any resources that would be helpful for us. There were plenty of pamphlets on breast cancer, prostate cancer, lung cancer, colon cancer, skin cancer, but none on urethral cancer.

Feeling a headache brewing, I rubbed my forehead, wondering where to go to find information on this type of cancer. Standing there in the middle of the room, I noticed a secretary typing speedily on her keyboard. *Well, I can find almost anything on the Internet.*

I turned around and saw Chris strutting down the hall, rubbing the Band-Aid on his arm, smiling.

"So, who's hungry, because I'm starved?"

I looked at him and laughed.   Only Chris would still have an appetite after all this.

During dinner, Mark and Toni asked Chris how he felt about Dr. Needles.

"I like him. I have a positive feeling that he'll be a good doctor for me." He looked around the table, "I have a good team," he said. "This cancer doesn't know who it's messing with. I'm going to beat this."

I leaned back and watched him with his family. He wasn't overwhelmed by this cancer. He was ready on his mark, anxious to begin his fight – his race. It reminded me of Chris' determination in the Labor Day bicycle race a couple of weeks before and how he kept an optimistic attitude despite its challenges.

28

Throughout the summer, Chris trained hard to prepare for the criterion race. He competed several times and had to be pulled out each time. This year, his goal was to finish the race.

We arrived early that morning so Chris could have plenty of time to preview the course and get ready. He was so focused that he barely spoke. I gave him plenty of space while he stretched, warmed up, and did a final check on his bike – a professional road bike made of light carbon steel that allows the rider to increase their speed, slice around the corners, and easily pedal with a steady cadence.

"Good luck," I told him and watched him pedal off on his bright red, black, and white bicycle. He chose to wear one of his favorite jerseys in bold red, orange, yellow, black and white that showed off his biceps. Waiting for the people to pass by, I noticed how his long, muscular legs moved gracefully, clicking his shoe into the pedal and crossing the street.

When the race was about to begin, all the cyclists rode up to the starting line and got into position while everyone rang their cowbells for them. Someone was shouting directions to the cyclists in a microphone and I wondered if they could hear what was being said with all of the excitement. It was so crowded that I barely got close enough to see Chris. He found me, smiled and then bowed his head.

The starting gun echoed a loud *BANG!* and the cyclists clicked into their pedals and darted forward in one swift, choreographed movement. In a matter of seconds they rounded the corner and disappeared. About 10 minutes later, we saw them sprinting around the corner at the opposite end of the street and everyone started going crazy again. I squeezed my feet in between the poles of the barricade and stood up on my toes to look for Chris. I found him keeping up the pace in the middle of the group.

"Go Chris, go," I yelled.

They whisked by and I felt the wind blow on my face. With wide eyes, I shivered, feeling the energy flow through my body, making me want to get on a bike and join them.

After the third lap, the cyclists still had a lot of energy and the race was getting more intense. There was a small group of riders several feet ahead of the rest of the pack. I gripped the fence, looking for Chris and found him at the back of the larger group.

"Come on Chris, you can do it! Ride hard," I shouted.

This time, the wait seemed more like a half-an-hour rather than just several minutes longer. I kept checking my watch, bouncing my foot and tapping my fingers.

"Here they come for the fifth lap," the announcer bellowed. The riders flew past us so quickly, it was all a blur. Not too far behind, there was a smaller group of cyclists pedaling hard. I found Chris' jersey in the lead.

"Come on guys, let's do it!" Chris yelled out and everyone rang their cowbells to cheer them on.

Sometime during the lap, the riders in Chris' group separated. They veered around the corner, one by one, riding on their own and falling further behind. I wondered why they didn't stay together, but Chris kept his head down and pedaled harder.

"Keep going, Chris. Stay strong. You can do it," I screamed.

He pushed himself off his seat, sprinted and turned the corner for the sixth time. I had no idea what it took to endure this kind of race and admired his perseverance.

Toward the end of the lap, Chris and the other cyclists were too far behind and had to be pulled out of the race. He dropped his head over the handlebars and slowly steered off the course. I could only imagine how disappointed he must have felt. He tried so hard. I left the race and waited for him by his truck. Eventually, I saw him pull into the parking lot. He stopped in front of me, took off his helmet, riding gloves, and sunglasses, and then kissed me.

"I'm proud of you, Chris. You're a winner to me."

"Thanks babe," he smiled, wiping the sweat from his forehead.

After Chris loaded up his bike and changed, we watched the race winding down to the final laps.

"Steph, this was the best I've ever done. Last year, it was at the end of the fourth lap when I got pulled out. I rode two more laps. Next year, I'm going to finish this race."

"I believe you will, Chris."

Mark's boisterous laugh brought me back to their conversation. I looked at my fiancé' and felt his confidence. *Yes, I believe you will beat this cancer, Chris.*

Get Set

"...for in You alone I put my trust. Show me the way I should walk."

- Psalm 143:8

Chris juggled the three tests around his work schedule while I worked and searched the Internet sites about urethral cancer. I needed to understand what we were dealing with and how we could fight it together. I learned that there were about 500 documented cases with only a few of the cancer centers in the country having had some experience in dealing with this type of cancer with no consensus on how to treat it. While I understood very little of what I read, what I did grasp was this: Chris had cancer – a rare form of cancer. According to the website, our only options were watchful waiting, surgery, chemotherapy, or radiation therapy. But which method do we use to fight it?

I stared at the computer screen and felt a heaviness fill my chest. I had hoped to find answers. Instead I discovered what rare meant in the medical field and was getting discouraged. *How do I explain all of this to Chris without sounding hopeless and worried? Oh God, show me what to do?* I pulled out my Bible and God guided me on what to do through His Word.

"The Lord is near. Do not be anxious about anything. In everything resort to prayer and supplication together with thanksgiving and bring your requests before God. Then the peace of God, which surpasses all understanding, will keep your hearts and minds in Christ Jesus."

- Philippians 4:5 – 7

After reading this scripture, I felt a sense of peace taking away the heavy weight. I realized that I was not supposed to handle this by myself and I prayed. *God, You know what to do, so I will put my faith and hope in You. Show me how to support Chris in the way he needs me.*

After what felt like a month, the follow-up appointment finally came. We found out there was just the one tumor located within the lining of the urethra, which meant the cancer was in the first stage. *Thank you, God.*

"We have a good chance to control the cancer before any other cells formed more tumors," Dr. Needles said. "I think we should try chemotherapy first rather than surgery to remove the tumor. If we could find the right chemo, not only would it destroy the tumor itself but the cancer cells as well," he suggested.

"I'll do whatever it takes to fight this thing," Chris said.

Dr. Needles recommended Cisplatin and Gemzar. He wanted to do the chemo once a day over a three-week period and give Chris a week off before the next round. He hoped to do three rounds and then get another MRI.

"Doctor, can I do chemo everyday?" Chris asked.

We learned that the chemo drugs were so potent that it could kill him if we did it daily. I stared at the doctor with wide eyes. *What is he prescribing for Chris?*

"We will check your red blood cell and white blood cell counts before each treatment to make sure your body can endure it," Dr. Needles explained. "We will assess the side effects you might experience such as fatigue, fever, nausea, vomiting, diarrhea, and loss of appetite. You may also have delayed side effects such as ringing in the ears and the feeling of numbness and tingling in your fingers and toes." My hand shook while I tried to write all of this in our notebook. *This is too much. How can one begin to fathom all of this and still want to go through it?*

"No problem. I can handle it," Chris said confidently. I stopped and looked at him, surprised. Dr. Needles wrote out the orders and asked if we had any questions.

"Yes, I have a question," Chris piped up. "When can I get back on my bike?"

I held my breath.

"Chris," Dr. Needles paused, "you can do all the normal physical activities *except* bike riding because I'm afraid it might aggravate the tumor."

Chris pressed his lips together, leaned back in his chair, and rubbed the side of his forehead.

"Okay. It's only temporary. I'll be back riding soon," he said optimistically. Dr. Needles handed the orders to Chris and paused again, facing the both of us.

"Do you plan to have children?" he asked.

What? Where is he going with this? Chris squeezed my hand.

"We hoped to start trying after getting married," he told Dr. Needles.

"Okay," he nodded, "but the only way you would be able to do this is if you banked the sperm before starting chemo treatment," Dr. Needles said, looking at Chris.

I didn't know what to say. I just sat there. Chris glanced at me with so much love in his eyes, squeezed my hand, and smiled. When I didn't think it was possible to fall deeper in love with this man, he would say or do something that would amaze me. Dr. Needles suggested an infertility and reproductive clinic for us to go to and gave him the information. Chris had time to take care of this since he couldn't start chemo until the insurance company approved it. Dr. Needles thought a week should be a sufficient amount of time and scheduled the treatment during the first week in October.

However, there were limited openings at the clinic. The only appointment that was available was during Chris' lunch break the day before he was supposed to start chemo.

When Chris called me that evening, he didn't sound like he was in a good mood.

"Hey babe, how was your day with the kids?" he asked. I really wanted to know about his day, but I could tell he didn't want to talk. I babbled on about my lessons and my students. It wasn't like him to be so quiet.

"Chris, what's wrong?" I finally asked.

"Steph, I had a terrible day. I went to the clinic and they didn't have the report that was supposed to have been faxed from the Air Guard, since I recently had a complete physical exam from them. I couldn't get anyone there during the lunch hour, so I drove to the office at the airport to get another copy. By then, I had to get back to work. When my shift ended, I went back to the clinic and the office was already closed. I missed it by 10 minutes. Can you believe it? I'm sorry, Steph. I feel like I've let you down," he said.

"Chris, listen, it's not your fault. I can't imagine you ever letting me down and I don't want you to worry about that anymore. Okay?" I said, trying to comfort him.

"Thanks."

Then I realized Chris was supposed to start chemo the next day. I couldn't believe at the bad timing.

"Uh, Chris, you're supposed to start chemo tomorrow."

"I know."

"Well, maybe you can reschedule it for Friday and get into the clinic..."

"No, Steph. I'm not waiting another day," Chris said firmly.

I tried to rationalize that it was just one more day.

"Steph, I feel like I've waited too long already. I need to do something now," he yelled. "I have cancer! I can't stand that it is in my body and I have no way to get it out. I can't live one more day waiting and doing nothing. Do you understand? I need to start this fight now."

I could hear the frustration in his voice while I sat there on the couch, crying. What could I say? I couldn't imagine having cancer – an invasion that threatened to attack his body and destroy everything he had worked so hard for, for so long. Ever since Chris was a young boy, he had always taken good care of himself. Even under peer pressure, he wouldn't do anything that could put him or anyone else in danger.

Chris was around 9-years-old when he and his mother lived in Wisconsin where he especially loved the cold weather. One time, he and a friend wanted to go sledding and came upon a steep hill. They talked about how thrilling it would be to slide down it. However, there was a small pond at the bottom with trees surrounding it, and Chris wasn't sure if it was completely frozen since it was still early in the season. Even if it was, he figured there wouldn't be enough room to stop and worried they might crash into the trees. His friend dared Chris to do it with him. But Chris refused, telling his friend he had a strange feeling they shouldn't ride down this hill. But he shrugged Chris off as he jumped onto his sled and speedily descended down the hill. He lost his balance, tumbled out of the sled, slid across the pond, and then landed upside down in the middle of the frozen pond. When his friend didn't move right away, Chris stood there in horror thinking his friend might have broken his neck or his back, or worse, he was dead. A man appeared and yelled at them, demanding to know what they were up to. After several long minutes, his friend came to, stood up, and ran away. Chris turned around and made his way back home. He was relieved his friend was okay, but it left Chris shaken. He thought it was such a stupid and reckless dare. His friend could have fallen through the ice, become paralyzed, or he could have been killed. Chris thought how devastating it would be to never be able to move, walk, run, or ride a bike – to always be in a prison of immobility. He asked God not to let that happen to him and made a promise he wouldn't do anything that could jeopardize his body or his health.

I knew Chris would never risk his life or our future. I couldn't grasp how it felt to deal with cancer inside your body. How could I tell him that I understood? How could I change his mind to wait one more day as anxious as he was to begin his fight?

"Don't worry, Steph, it'll all work out," Chris said. I wasn't so sure when I hung up the phone, still feeling confused and defeated.

I did the only thing I was certain about – I prayed.

God, you know that it is in our hearts to have a baby together. I want to do what's best for Chris and I also want to do what would be best for us, too. I'm torn on what is the right thing to do, so I'm turning to you with hope. If it is meant for us to have a family, I believe you will make it happen.

Go!

"Get on with it. Start running – never quit! Keep your eyes on Jesus, who both began and finished this race."

- Hebrews 12:1, 2

I met Chris at his house so we could go to the cancer center together.

"Good morning. How's my girl?"

I smiled nervously and hugged him tightly.

"No worries," he whispered and kissed my forehead. He had such a great attitude. I thought maybe he was right and I shouldn't worry so much.

After we arrived at the cancer center, Chris went to the lab for blood work then signed in at Dr. Needles' office. We didn't have to wait long and he remembered the routine to check his vitals which were all normal and he weighed in at 170 pounds. We found out that the insurance company approved the treatment and Chris' blood work was excellent. He was off to a good start.

Taking the chemo order from Dr. Needles, he was ready, but I squeezed his hand to keep him from standing up. He glanced at me, squeezed back, and then talked about the problems he had and how he wasn't able to bank the sperm. Dr. Needles explained that if Chris chose to start this treatment, it would be a risk, but it might still be okay after the first round of chemo. He would need to have a few weeks of rest to allow his body to recuperate before trying again.

I clenched my jaws and tried to breathe normally. *What's one more day? Oh God, please.* Chris leaned back in his chair quietly and I felt a glimmer of hope that he was going to change his mind.

"Steph, I really need to get started on my fight."

This is not what I wanted to hear.

Dr. Needles left the room silently. I packed up our notebook, keeping my head down, and fighting back the tears. Chris slung the backpack over his shoulder, pulled me close to him and lifted my chin.

"Steph, I really believe it will all work out for us and I want you to believe too," he whispered. I laid my head on his shoulder and hugged him tightly. *God, I hope he's right. You know our dream of having a family.*

"This is what Yahweh says, 'For I know what my plans for you are, plans to save you and not to harm you, plans to give you a future and to give you hope.'"

- Jeremiah 29:11

I didn't have time to regroup when we walked into the treatment room. Nothing could have prepared me for what I saw. I tried not to look shocked and pressed my lips together. The room was already busy with patients hooked up to IV's and most of them were much older than Chris. I couldn't believe that there were seniors fighting cancer. It didn't seem right to me. They lived many years working hard and caring for their families. They should be enjoying their retirement, not spending it in a cancer center. Some of them looked solemn and pale, weak and worn out, and so thin and fragile. Several were wearing hats or scarves and were wrapped tightly in warm blankets. I didn't know what to think or how to feel for them, for Chris, or for myself. But Chris hadn't noticed. He was preoccupied on deciding which recliner looked the most comfortable, picked the one he wanted and settled into it. I took a deep breath to calm my nerves. He smiled that goofy grin of his and patted the armrest.

"Wanna sit here next to me, sweetheart?" he asked, impersonating Humphrey Bogart's voice. "I promise *not* to behave," he winked.

Before I could respond, a nurse came over and began telling us about the treatment Chris was about to endure over the next six hours. We found out Cisplatin can cause kidney damage and Chris would get fluids to flush his kidneys while receiving this drug. Then he would need to drink about two quarts or more of liquids at home over the next 24 hours. Gemzar would take about an hour and was somewhat less potent. Both chemo drugs were known to cause a loss of appetite, fatigue, and a drop in blood cell counts. Chris was advised to stay away from his favorite foods during the treatments because later he would not be able to enjoy them anymore. She stressed that should he have a 101 degree-fever or higher, vomiting, or diarrhea to call the office right away. When I took the information cards from the nurse, it felt like a heavy weight had been put in my hands. *Oh my God, what are we getting ourselves into with all of this?*

"Are you ready to get started Chris?" the nurse asked.

He winked at me again, looked at his nurse and responded in his best Austrian accent,

"I'm ready [clap] to be [clap] pumped up [clap, clap, snap, snap]," and gave both thumbs up. Laughing, I just shook my head at him.

She stared at him with wide eyes.

"Trust me, you will be pumped up," she said dryly.

I turned to her sharply, but it didn't faze Chris at all. She started his IV and I watched the transparent liquid flow from the bag through the tube and finally into its destination: my fiancé's body. I felt sick to my stomach, swallowing hard to keep my breakfast down. *Could this really be happening?*

We were putting a dangerous chemical into Chris' body – poison to kill the tumor and cancer cells that also lowers blood cell counts he would need to fight off an infection and to stay healthy. It was all backwards to me. Medicine was created to heal the body, not destroy it. It was almost more than I could bear to watch. I bowed my head, closed my eyes, and prayed. *God, let this treatment destroy the evil that is lurking in this man's body.*

Suddenly I felt pressure on my hand and looked up at Chris. Unbelievably, he was smiling at me.

"No worries," he said confidently. I couldn't find my voice. I swallowed down the lump in my throat and smiled back at him.

We watched a video that gave us an overview about chemotherapy. I learned that we would need to adjust Chris' diet to foods rich in antioxidants, iron, protein, and carbohydrates. He would need to slow down on his physical activities to allow more time to rest and recover from the chemo treatment. *Yeah right. Easier said than done with him.* I glanced at Chris, wondering what he was thinking about this, but he was already sleeping. The nurse came by to check his IV and told me that she had given him a dose of Benadryl to help him relax and to bypass any nauseating sensations he might feel during the chemo. I carefully took off his head phones and let him rest.

The day crept along slowly. I saw patients come and go. At one point, it was so busy that every chair was occupied and a couple of people had to wait. *Just how many people are afflicted with cancer?* But no one complained. I realized that I hadn't heard a negative word all day. I felt the strength, determination and hope from everyone – patients, caregivers, nurses, doctors, and office personnel – and I began to admire them for their courage and perseverance.

I reviewed the research information and notes from our meetings with Dr. Needles and wondered how Chris and I could fight against this kind of cancer? I shivered and took another deep breath. Just then, I knew – deep within me – what we had to do. We must truly believe in our faith and trust God, hope for healing, and love each other and God throughout this race. For it says,

"...love believes all things, hopes all things, endures all things. Love will never end."

– 1st Corinthians 13:7 – 8

From the moment Chris and I met, we experienced so much joy and love beyond what we could ever hope for. Even with the diagnosis, we were still very happy and deeply in love with one another – and we knew God was there with us.

"[Jesus said,] as the Father has loved me, so I have loved you; remain in my love. I have told you all this, that my own joy may be in you and your joy may be complete. This is my commandment: love one another as I have loved you."

– John 15:9, 11 – 12

It was around 3 p.m. when the treatment was over and Chris woke up, bursting with energy.

"I'm starving," he clapped his hands. "What do you want to do for dinner?"

I laughed but was glad he had an appetite after all of that chemo. We decided on BBQ take-out and took it back to his place. Soon after we ate, Chris began to feel tired and wanted to turn in early. I kissed him goodbye and left wondering if he would have any side effects throughout the night. I wished I could stay to watch over him, but I had to go home to take care of my dogs and prepare to return to school the next day. It took every bit of energy I had left to drive away and I finally let the tears go. *Oh God, watch over Chris for me. Protect him.*

Over the weekend, Chris started feeling some of the side effects: fatigue, tightness in his stomach, and ringing in his ears which really annoyed him. However, through the week, his appetite gradually returned back to normal and he started getting some of his energy back. Chris continued to work at the casino supervising the security personnel and enforcing gaming regulations. I didn't have to worry about him working on the road in the different weather conditions or dealing with traffic and accidents.

Early one morning, Chris noticed that the tumor felt softer and he called me right away. We felt more optimistic and hopeful this treatment was working and thanked God for this good sign. By Friday, the ringing in his ears had faded some and he lost two pounds. Chris' blood count was stable and he was able to do another hour of Gemzar.

On the third week, we ran into a roadblock and found out that Chris' white blood cell counts were too low to do the third hour of Gemzar. Dr. Needles suggested using this as a week off and to begin the second round the following week with both drugs.

"It's all good," Chris said, unfazed by this setback.

During the break, Chris regained his physical strength and ate more protein and carbohydrates to gain back his weight. He kept his promise to me and went back to the infertility clinic to take care of our future the day before the next round of chemo.

Chris' blood work was normal and he gained more than four pounds, weighing in at 172 pounds. I stayed by his side again during the long six-hour treatment. He slept while I observed the steady drip of the chemo pumping through the IV into Chris' vein. I buried my head in my hands and felt the warm, salty tears flow into them. I hated watching Chris and other patients endure this battle. I hated the chemo and the side effects it caused. I hated cancer. Finally, I got out my Bible, hoping to find strength and reassurance from God in all of this. After skimming through it, I was led to a scripture from Deuteronomy 31:8,

"The Lord himself goes before you and will be with you; He will never leave you nor forsake you. Do not be afraid; do not be discouraged."

I don't know how I got there, but once I read those words, I knew they were for me at that very moment. I leaned back in my chair, closed my eyes and envisioned Jesus sitting between us and holding us in the palm of his hands. He was encouraging us to be strong and not to be afraid, and he would always be with us. I took several long deep breaths and felt a surreal kind of peace fill my heart. I almost dozed off but was alerted by a constant, annoying beeping from an IV machine. I checked on Chris and saw he was fine, still napping. *That has to be some powerful Benadryl.*

Relieved, I looked around to figure out what was going on. But it was the same scenario: most patients were elderly with a few around Chris' age fighting for their lives. Despite the gruesome task of the nurses giving chemotherapy and the patients receiving it, everyone stayed positive and optimistic. Giving up was not an option – there was always hope.

I reread the scripture and prayed. I began to feel courage deep within me unlike anything I had felt before. I knew I could keep going in this fight as long as I trusted God to help Chris and me through it. Looking at my fiancé, I realized this what Chris had been feeling all along.

Over the next several days, the side effects from the drugs hit Chris harder. He didn't have a lot of energy and took several naps. His appetite was poor – nothing smelled or tasted good to him. I cooked several homemade meals to entice him with savoring smells in his house, but he couldn't eat more than several bites. Chris lost three pounds that week, but his blood counts remained stable and he endured another hour of Gemzar. By the beginning of the following week, the ringing in his ears faded, his appetite improved, and he began to feel more energy again. We were starting to see a pattern of what to expect after each chemo treatment. However, Chris didn't experience pain from the tumor anymore. He was getting more anxious to keep up with the chemo, despite the side effects.

Expecting to get the third hour of Gemzar, we hit the same roadblock again – Chris' white blood cell count was too low. Dr. Needles suggested stopping the treatment to check the status of the tumor and ordered another round of tests: MRI, CT-Scan, and a PET-Scan. Chris wasn't deterred.

"It's all good," he told me.

Walking out of the cancer center into the sun's golden light, I felt its warmth comforting me. It was as if I was feeling God's loving hands stroking my face, reminding me, *I am here.*

Soar High

"...those who hope in Yahweh will renew their strength. They will soar as with eagle's wings."

- Isaiah 40:31

After a week of tests, we couldn't wait to hear the good news. My notebook was opened and my pen ready, anxious to take notes when the door opened and Dr. Needles walked in quietly. He sat down on the stool at the desk and flipped Chris' file to a page and studied it. I tried to disguise the tight feeling of unease that suddenly crept into my chest, studying the doctor's every move, trying to find out something from his face, which remained irritatingly impassive. After several long seconds, I glanced at Chris, who was also watching his doctor. I held his hand when Dr. Needles finally faced us with a grim expression.

"The chemo has not been very effective against the tumor. It has grown bigger. However the intensity inside of it has decreased, meaning it is less active. Maybe that's why it felt softer and didn't cause any more discomfort for you," he said to Chris.

"Doctor, if it's less active then how did the tumor grow?" I asked bewildered, trying to make sense of this.

He shook his head, "I don't know. Cisplatin is a very potent drug but it wasn't enough to break down this tumor. This particular cancer consists of squamous cells, which is the most aggressive type to fight. I consulted with the doctors from several cancer centers again and they don't understand it either. I also brought Chris' case to a team of doctors here to review and brainstorm treatment options."

I struggled to stay calm. Before all of this, I thought there was only one kind of cancer but in different areas of the body. I had no idea that there were different types of cancerous cells and several stages of the cancer. Overwhelmed, I wondered what we could do to fight this particular cancer.

It felt like trying to find a needle in a haystack in which you keep looking and trying different strategies to find it but if you continue to search, there was a chance it could slip deeper into the haystack. Then you had to make a decision – keep looking or wait until you figure out a better strategy. Either way, it was a risk because you needed to find that needle sooner rather than later. This rare cancer was like that. Where could we look to find the answers – to find a cure – sooner rather than later?

I couldn't bear to look at Chris.

After several long minutes of silence, Dr. Needles continued, "Dr. Chehval is also on this team and we recommend surgery to remove the tumor in order to try to contain and control this cancer."

"If the tumor is inside the lining of the urethra, how will it be removed?" I asked.

"I'm not sure how aggressive the surgery would be. I'm not a surgeon, so you will need to discuss this with Dr. Chehval," he explained. "However, I am obliged to tell you that you can get another opinion."

Finally, I looked over at Chris who had been quietly listening and rubbing the side of his temple.

"No," he said forcefully, sitting up straighter. "I want to stay here. I feel like I'm where I'm supposed to be. I'll do whatever it takes to beat this thing," he said.

"Okay," said Dr. Needles. "The next step is to get an accurate measurement on the size of the tumor and the exact location of it in the urethra. We would also need to know if the bladder is clear of the cancer."

My eyes widened, "What? We have to worry about cancer in the bladder?" I blurted out. Chris squeezed my hand. I leaned back in my chair and pressed my lips together.

Dr. Needles continued, "Dr. Chehval wrote out an order for a CT-scan and an MRI of the bladder and of the urethra." He handed it to Chris. "Then you will meet with him to go over the results and discuss your options." He told us that the tests were already scheduled during the first week of December. I opened my calendar book and the weight bore down on my shoulders.

"That's about three weeks away," I said. 10 days of waiting was bad enough. Dr. Needles stood up and shook Chris' hand.

"Dr. Chehval will keep me informed. Good luck," then he turned and left the room quickly. We walked out quietly and passed by the receptionist without making a follow-up appointment, breaking our familiar routine. It felt like we had reached a dead-end that forced us to turn around and head back to the starting line. I imagined the tumor inside of Chris' body and shivered, feeling the goose bumps all over my arms and legs. I felt a tingling fear of this monster within the core of my body. Suddenly, Chris swept me around to face him.

"Steph, it's going to be okay," he said strongly.

"But how do you know, Chris?" I cried. "The doctors don't even know." He looked at the dreary clouds that fit perfectly with the sudden change of my mood.

"I just know. As long as there is hope, I will not give up."

I followed his gaze upward. *Okay God. We are not giving up.*

Later that night, I tossed and turned, thinking how we would get through the next 20 days. Surrendering to the useless battle to get some sleep, I sat up and turned on my lamp, grabbed my Bible from my nightstand and held it close to my heart. The strength and patience that we needed would have to come from God. I noticed a piece of paper sticking out from inside the front cover and pulled it out. It was an email from a friend with a scripture.

"You are my servant; I have chosen you and have not cast you away, fear not, for I am with you; be not dismayed, for I am your God, I will give you strength, I will bring you help."

- Isaiah 41: end of 9, 10

I felt God's comfort and strength through His words and I called Chris.

"I'm sorry to wake you, but I couldn't wait until morning to share this scripture I just read." I told him how I got it and read it to him. He was quiet for several seconds.

"Wow. That's awesome, Steph. How can I be afraid if God is on my side?" He laughed, "We're going to beat this together."

After a week of waiting, Chris gave me a letter that renewed my strength to get through another 13 days before we would see Dr. Chehval.

"Dear Stephanie, it is so very hard to find the words to describe how happy and how loved you make me feel. It's even more difficult to tell you how much I appreciate you. In my fight against cancer, you have been a bright star in a sea of darkness. I'm sorry that you have had to endure the sadness, stress and worry associated with this fight. I admire and appreciate your strength and courage to stand with me through all of this. Thank you for being here for me. Thank you for being my light.

The happiness of one's life is measured by those who have brought love and joy into it. And the happiness in my life, since meeting you, is immeasurable.

I love you. Chris."

I held his letter close to my heart and looked at a picture that was taken on the night Chris proposed. *What had I done to deserve this wonderful man who has brought so much more happiness in my life each day.* It was so appropriate to receive this letter during the Thanksgiving holiday. I thanked God for our families and friends and for bringing Chris into my life. I continued to pray for complete healing over this cancer and for the strength and grace to keep riding on with him without ever giving up hope.

Looking back at this turning part of our journey, I began to understand the deeper meaning of hope through God's Word and how He was there with us through our family, friends, and even strangers at the right moments when we needed Him the most.

Chris and I worked to develop a more meaningful relationship with Jesus by reading, discussing and learning, meditating, and praying over the scriptures passed on to us or those that just happened to come to our attention from looking through the Bible or listening to someone. It didn't happen overnight. It took us awhile, but Chris already knew without a doubt that God was with him in his race. Just like the strength of an eagle soaring high in the skies, without ever falling, Chris knew he could stay strong in his hope. The scripture from Isaiah 41:31 confirms this.

"...those who hope in Yahweh will renew their strength. They will soar as with eagle's wings; they will run and not grow weary; they will walk and never tire."

Resilience

"Giving up is one of the easiest things to do. But to hold it together when everyone else would understand if you fell apart, that's the true strength."

- Author Unknown

The day finally came to see Dr. Chehval. It felt like I had been on this route before. Usually when you travel on the same course, you begin to recognize certain things and know what to expect up ahead. But this path wasn't exactly the same and the outcome of it was definitely going to be different.

Throughout the day, I kept checking the time and willed it to tick faster. The distractions of teaching my lessons and working with my students helped pass the time. But when I had some quiet moments, I couldn't concentrate on my work. I kept wondering what Dr. Chehval would tell us. I stared out my window and watched the leafless trees sway in the wind. The one thing I dreaded most about the winter season was that life around you seemed to let go and get buried somewhere under the earth. I noticed hundreds of branches pointing in every imaginable direction from its trunk and wondered which direction this surgery would take us. How difficult would it be for Chris? Would it be successful to remove the cancer and cure him? I could feel my pulse pound against my temples, causing one of those annoying, lingering headaches. All of this waiting, not knowing, and the uncertainty of what Dr. Chehval would tell us was wearing me down. I still hadn't caught on how to let go of my worries and give them to God.

When the dismissal bell finally rang, I already had my purse and keys in my hand and I flew out of my classroom, not bothering to turn off the lights and locking my door. I passed by my astonished students who knew I would've corrected them if they were running down the stairs. But I didn't care. I just wanted to get to Chris as soon as possible.

Driving quickly on the highway, I had to remind myself to stay within the speed limit. I knew Chris would scowl if he knew I was driving like this. I found the tall office building and parked in the garage across from it. Chris was already waiting for me at the entrance when I ran up to him.

"We have plenty of time," he said, laughing while I caught my breath and shook my head, wondering how he could be so cool. He took my hand and led me inside. Once in the elevators, Chris pushed the button for the top floor and we waited quietly during the slow ride passing each floor at a time.

After signing in, we walked to the end of the hall, into Dr. Chehval's office and sat in the chairs before his massive mahogany desk piled with folders, papers, notes, and large manila envelopes with x-rays. I began to jiggle my leg and tapping my pen against our notebook. Chris put his hand over mine.

"Sorry," I whispered.

"It's going to be okay, Steph."

I took a deep breath and welcomed the distractions on the bookshelves against the wall behind the doctor's desk displaying many books, football memorabilia, certificates, awards, and photographs.

"Chris, look." I pointed out a sign on one shelf that read, *"Don't accept a drink from an Urologist!"* and we started laughing until the door suddenly opened. A man in a white lab coat with light gray hair walked in.

"Hello Chris," greeted Dr. Chehval and shook his hand. "How are you doing?"

Chris told him that he was doing well and then introduced me. He chatted with us for a few minutes, making us feel more at ease with him and then began to go over the test results.

"Of the two tests, the MRI was the best one to analyze on what to do. The good news is that the tumor is localized, which means no other tumors were found."

I grabbed Chris' hand. *Thank you, God.*

Dr. Chehval continued. "The tumor is located inside the lining of the urethra," he explained, showing us on a model that was on his desk, "and I suggest taking the least aggressive approach to remove it: that is to cut and remove part of the urethra where the tumor is located."

I studied the model. *Okay, but how would Chris relieve himself?*

As if he read my mind, he went on. "In doing this Chris, you will not be able to void normally. I would have to create an opening where you can be relieved by sitting. This is only temporary. After about four to six months, if everything looks good, I will do a urethral resection – which is a reconstructive surgery to repair the urethra that will allow you to void normally again." Dr. Chehval paused, giving us a moment to process all of this. Speechless, I sat there, trying to understand just how much of Chris' lifestyle would change.

"The surgery should take about two hours and you would be in the hospital at least two days for observation. You would need to use a catheter for awhile to allow your body to recover and then you should be able to void on your own."

Dr. Chehval folded his hands on his desk and waited. I rubbed my forehead, trying to make sense of everything. Chris was stiff as a board and kept nodding. He let go of my hand to put his elbows on his knees and leaned forward.

"Can I do radiation since there is only one tumor?" he asked.

"In the team meeting, Dr. Needles talked about the possibility of doing radiation. However, the radiologists strongly believed that it would not work since chemotherapy didn't shrink the tumor," Dr. Cheval paused. "They don't want to put you through the painful effects of radiation since the tumor is located just under the skin. The burns from it would be excruciatingly unbearable for you, Chris."

Oh my God!

My heart was pounding so hard that I was sure it echoed in the room, but no one seemed to notice. I looked at my notebook on my lap and saw that I hadn't written a single word, but gripping the pen as if my life depended on it. I knew if I looked at Chris again, I'd lose it so I started taking notes.

"Chris, this doesn't just affect you, but Stephanie as well since you will be getting married in June." I stopped in the middle of a word and looked at the doctor. He continued.

"I also want you to know that you can get another opinion. You have a lot to think about and I recommend that the both of you talk it over before making a decision," he said.

At that moment, I realized that cancer doesn't just attack the patient – it throws daggers at their caregivers and loved ones closest to him or her. I had just a little bit of courage left in me to look over at Chris and he nodded.

"Okay," Dr. Chehval said. "Take a couple of days to think about this before letting me know what you decide. Do you have any questions?"

"Yes, I do," Chris answered optimistically. "How soon can I get back on my bike?"

Stunned, I stared at Chris. Here I was, worried about the effects of the surgery and how it would change his life, but he was looking ahead, determined to beat this cancer and get back on his bike.

"Keep your sight on what is ahead and your eyes directed straight in front of you."

- Proverbs 4:25

I closed my mouth and turned to the doctor, fearful of what his answer might be and how Chris would react.

"I know you want to ride again Chris, but I'm afraid it might aggravate the tumor. I think you should stay off the bike until about a month after the surgery, but it could be longer depending on your recovery. If you want to exercise, you may be able to walk on the treadmill about two to three weeks after the surgery."

Chris pressed his lips together, sat back in the chair, crossed his arms over his chest and began rubbing the side of his temple. My shoulders dropped, feeling his disappointment. *How much does he have to sacrifice in order to fight this cancer?*

After we left Dr. Chehval's office, Chris wanted to go out to eat. I was relieved that his appetite was getting back to normal, but I couldn't imagine having dinner. I replayed the meeting over in my mind. Would Chris be strong enough to endure the changes in his body from this surgery? Was I strong enough to be there for him in the way he would need me? How could we prepare for all of this? If these thoughts were running through my mind, I wondered what was going on with Chris.

"What do you think about what Dr. Chehval told us?" I blurted out, breaking the silence.

He sighed, "I'm trying to process it all."

I studied my plate for awhile, waiting for Chris until he was ready to talk. I knew he needed some time to work it out. I took several more bites of my meal but struggled to swallow it. Giving up, I sat back and wondered if we should take Dr. Needles and Dr. Chehval's advice.

"Chris, have you thought about getting another opinion?" He shook his head.

"No, I don't want to go to another doctor. I feel comfortable with Dr. Chehval and I respect his opinion."

"But maybe we should..."

"Steph," Chris interrupted, "I trust him with my life. I don't want any other doctor operating on me but him." He was so determined and confident in his decision that I realized once Chris made up his mind, it would be difficult to convince him otherwise.

"Okay. Then we need to talk about this surgery," I whispered.

He looked a little uncomfortable and suddenly, he dropped his fork down on his plate. "I tried chemo and it didn't even shrink it," he said angrily. "I can't believe what I went through didn't make any impact on it at all. I want to do the surgery to remove it and get on with my life, our lives," he paused, "and I want to get back on my bike again."

I couldn't imagine all the emotions he must have felt enduring the physical challenges from the cancer within his body and being so limited from all the things he wanted to do. I reached across the table and held his hand. I didn't want to bring up the effect of the surgery, but it was unavoidable.

"Chris, do you understand how you'd have to do some things differently after this surgery?" I asked cautiously.

He pressed his lips tightly.

"It won't be so bad and it would only be for a few months," I said, trying to sound encouraging. "Tell you what, Chris. No one needs to know the details of the surgery. We can focus on telling our families and close friends that the tumor will be removed. We'll keep the specifics between us and your doctors. Okay?"

Looking relieved, he nodded. "I can handle that. But whatever happens, I will deal with it one day at a time. I'll do anything I have to do to fight this. Whatever it takes, I'm going to do it and I will beat this thing."

"But Chris, this isn't like when you were a kid. You don't have to fight alone," I whispered, thinking of the story he told me when he had to deal with a lot on his own.

When Chris was in his early teens, he and his mother finally adjusted to a fixed income and she was attending night school. Between her job and school, Chris treasured those special times they spent together, usually watching old black and white movies on the television. That is until she started dating again and eventually introduced Chris to a man she had been seeing.

Chris wasn't sure about him at first, but Phil made an effort to get to know him. He played basketball with him, took him to different places, and watched movies with him. To Chris, he seemed like a positive father-figure and it became the happiest time in his life.

However, everything changed when Phil and his mother got serious and he was spending more time at their apartment. Phil became verbally abusive to Chris whenever his mother wasn't around. The only time Phil was nice was when Chris' mother was present. He wanted to tell her what was going on, but he was afraid that she wouldn't believe him.

Chris learned that the best way to survive was to stay out of Phil's sight whenever he was around. Chris became engrossed with military aircraft and began building military airplane models, finding joy and a sense of accomplishment in a finished piece, especially those without any errors. The pleasure was short-lived because whatever made Chris happy, Phil would find a way to crush it. He limited the number of models Chris could buy even though he bought them with his own money. So, Chris started storing his models at one of his friend's house while keeping a few in his room. Several times, he was caught with too many kits or models according to Phil's rule – which would often change – and he would destroy them. But it didn't stop Chris from replacing the models, finding new joy improving his skills, and feeling the satisfaction of a much better finished product.

Eventually, Phil showed his true feelings toward Chris in front of his mother. One horrifying moment came when Chris saw Phil slap his mother after she tried to stop him from hurting Chris. He tried to help her, but she yelled at him to go to his room. Seeing the anger in her eyes, he quickly retreated to his bedroom and paced around, listening to more shouts. Suddenly, he heard the front door slam and all was quiet. Before Chris had a chance to figure out what to do, his door burst open and Phil flew in. He grabbed Chris, threw him on the floor, and held a large butcher knife to his throat.

"How *dare* you butt in my business? If you ever get in my way again, I'll kill you! Get out of here, you little bastard."

Chris scrambled away from Phil and ran out of the apartment with tears blurring his vision and fear making his entire body tremble. He didn't make it out of the garage of the apartment building and his mother somehow found him in the corner, hugging his knees tightly, crying. She held Chris and told him how sorry she felt for leaving him behind.

Chris dealt with so much on his own. He refused to give up and found strength within his spirit to keep on going and survived.

Sitting across from my fiancé, I could see the determination in his eyes. I squeezed his hand again, feeling so much love and admiration for him.

"Chris, you don't have to go through this by yourself," I reminded him again.

He looked down at his plate.

"Look at me," I said firmly. "You are *not* alone. I'm right here. We'll fight this cancer and beat it together. Chris, I'll always be by your side. I love you," I choked.

He studied me for a few seconds, then smiled sweetly and squeezed my hand.

"Thank you. I honestly don't think I can go through this without you. I love you so much."

We talked about the surgery and agreed to go ahead with it.

Chris called Dr. Chehval's office the next morning and found out that the surgery was scheduled for the following week. I thanked God we didn't have to wait long. I continued to pray for Chris and for Dr. Chehval that this surgery would be successful and Chris would be cancer-free.

Fear

"There is no fear in love."

- 1st John 4:18

Sometimes when you let your guard down or when you least expect it, fear can sneak into your heart and mind like a snake slithering in on its prey.

Saturday, before the surgery, Chris and I were relaxing together on the couch in his living room, watching a movie when I felt his arms close around me tightly. He buried his head in the curve of my neck and I felt warm, wet droplets sliding down to my shoulders. I couldn't imagine what was wrong. I turned around and wiped the salty tears from his cheeks. I waited silently for him to calm down, stroking his face. Finally he met my eyes.

"Steph, I'm scared." He squeezed me again and I held him for a long time.

"Chris, you're not alone. I'm here." I prayed for the words to comfort him, trying to be strong for him.

"I don't want you to be sad when I'm gone," he whispered.

I froze.

It was as if someone punched me in the middle of my chest and I couldn't breathe. I recognized this pain – the kind of agony that snuck in during the dark of the night like a thief. I experienced this once before and had hoped to never feel it again. It was fear.

When I was in my twenties, I met a guy and we hit it off right away. We were attracted to each other and flirted, but I would never let it get too far. I didn't want to have sex and I made sure he knew how I felt about it. But one night he persisted.

"No. I don't want to do this," I said, pushing him away. He ignored me.

"Stop it," I told him, "you know I don't want to..." and he smothered his mouth over mine. I tried to get away from him, but he pinned my hands under my back and put all his weight on top of me. I wiggled back and forth and tried to kick him, somehow he kept me down. The next thing I knew, he was forcing himself inside me. *Oh my God, I don't want to do this!* Panicking, I fought harder. I squirmed and twisted

53

to free my hands and legs. He was so much stronger. I still couldn't yell out, so I screamed in my mind, *"God, help me!"*

I opened my eyes and saw a figure that looked like a knight in a shining white armor on a white horse galloping through the door and I was suddenly freed from my attacker's hold. It was as if he was pulled off of me with such force that he shook his head like he was stunned and looked around. Backing away from him, I checked the door and there was no one there. I didn't care how or what just happened, I was relieved that the nightmare was over.

But the nightmare had only just begun. I felt lost inside. I didn't feel safe, secure, hopeful, or even loved anymore. I doubted that I would ever be whole or happy again. I didn't know who I was, what I was and what I was supposed to do with my life. I had no self-esteem or self-confidence. It felt like there was no sunshine in my heart, only dark, heavy clouds day after day. I was constantly nervous and anxious, checking over my shoulder and the activity around me. There were days when I had no strength and felt knocked down.

I was unsure about everything and had a difficult time making a decision – even over mundane things like what to eat for breakfast. I questioned myself all the time, most especially my instincts and trust of others – especially men. I wore a mask to hide what I was feeling from everyone, always looking over my shoulder and keeping my guard up. After several months, I knew I couldn't live like this any longer. I wanted to escape and start all over in a different place where no one knew me. I could be someone else with a new identity, someone who didn't wake up with a heavy burden, live all day in fear, and cry herself to sleep every night. I began to feel a glimpse of hope and thought maybe this was what I needed to do to move on.

When it felt like a door was closed, God would find a way to open another door. That was what happened one day when two close friends called me.

"We have this feeling that we should spend the afternoon together, so come on over," they said. I thought it was kind of odd and almost made an excuse not to come.

"Okay, I'm on my way," I blurted. We ended up talking all afternoon and for the first time in months, I laughed. I was amazed how good it felt. They helped me realize that if I could laugh again, then I could heal and put my life back together.

When I left, I noticed the summer's golden sun peeking through the trees against the deep blue sky and felt its warmth on my face. I started feeling some of the burden lift off my shoulders and I smiled. I felt this joy deep within my core rise up through my chest and out on my lips. It was hope and renewed strength.

I discovered a scripture that showed God's mercy on me at that moment. In Micah 7:8 – 9, it reads,

"Though I have fallen, I will rise. Though I sit in darkness, the Lord will be my light...He will bring me out into the light; I will see his righteousness."

This scripture described exactly what I'd been through and how I felt coming out of it, into the light of the sun – which to me was God's saving grace and love.

Looking back, I learned how God was there for me through my family and closest friends during what was the hardest time of my life. For it says,

"Be valiant and strong, do not fear or tremble... for Yahweh, your God is with you; He will not leave you or abandon you."

- Deuteronomy 31:6 and Joshua 1:9

Slowly, I began to re-discover who I was. I figured out what I wanted in my life and what I needed in a relationship with a man. I learned how to listen and follow my instincts – which I realized was my spirit. Little did I know then how important it was for me to figure this out before I met Chris so that I could be there for him in the way he would need me.

I refused to let this kind of fear attack Chris, and prayed for strength.

"Are you...? You're not..." I struggled to get the words out. I cleared my throat. "Chris, you're not giving up, are you?"

"No," he said with a shocked expression.

I looked at him questioningly.

"No, Steph. I'm fighting this thing. I'm not giving up. Now that you're a part of my life, I want to make you happy, as happy as you make me feel whenever I'm with you or think about you." I wiped his tears away and we held each other a long time.

"I am worried that you'll be so sad when I'm gone," he whispered in my ear.

The thought of Chris dying from this had never crossed my mind. The fear I felt about this cancer didn't compare to the fear I felt during the worst moment of my life years before. I couldn't bear the thought of losing him. *We finally found each other after all this time, surely God wouldn't let this cancer separate us now?* I couldn't believe this. *No!* I refused to believe it.

"Chris, are you thinking you may not be able to beat this cancer?"

"I don't know. I'm just scared, Steph." I prayed for guidance for the right words to say while I held him in my arms.

"I'm scared too. You're dealing with something that is threatening your life. But we're not going to let this cancer put fear into our relationship or in our faith in God. Chris, I love you so much. I will always be by your side and no matter what happens, we will beat this together." Chris started crying again and I held him fiercely, afraid to let him go, hoping he could feel my strength.

"I love you too, Steph." I dried his tears and he looked at me with a new spark in his eyes. "I'm not going to give up. I'm going to keep fighting and beat this thing."

I thanked God for being there for us.

"My flesh and my heart may fail, but God is the strength of my heart and my portion forever."

- Psalm 73:26

I often wondered about that knight who rescued me. It was real – as real in my mind today as it was at that critical moment. I still don't know why this happened, but I truly believe God sent one of his angels to help me. For it says,

"Say to those who are afraid: 'Have courage, do not fear. See, your God comes, demanding justice. He is the God who comes to save you.'"

- Isaiah 35:4

While Chris and I were dating, I told him what had happened to me. In his response, he held me close to him and said,

"I promise you, Steph, to always be there for you, to love you, and to protect you."

It was this incredible act of love from God through Chris that finally and completely healed me many years later.

"There is no fear in love. Perfect love drives away fear."

- 1st John 4:18

No Worries!

"Place all your worries on Him since He takes care of you."
- 1 Peter 5:7

Chris and I arrived about a half-an-hour early at the surgery center. I kept checking on him to make sure he was doing okay. He'd catch my eye and smile. I heard a long, low growling sound. Chris shook his head, leaned against the wall behind him, folded his arms across his stomach and closed his eyes. I tried to pay attention to the morning news on television but I couldn't help noticing how many people were there and wondered how many surgeries they could schedule at once. It seemed like we sat there a long time when we finally heard a lady call out Chris' name. We followed her into one of the prep rooms where he changed into a hideous faded gray hospital gown with bright blue footies over his socks. When he stepped out of the bathroom, the gown was just above his knees. I raised my eyebrows at him.

"Woohoo, Chris, you do have sexy legs," I said, fanning myself. "Do you want me to tie the strings together in the back for you?" Laughing, he shook his head.

"I already got it covered, babe."

"Hmmm, maybe I should check to make sure," I winked. "Really, I don't mind."

"Oh, behave!" he said, wagging his finger at me. He sat on the hospital bed and bounced his feet back and forth with a goofy grin, creating other voices for his feet as if they were having their own conversation.

"You are not right Chris," I said, laughing.

A new nurse knocked on the door and came in with a maroon binder with Chris' name on it and began the first of many question and answer interviews.

"What is your birth date? What are your allergies? Do you wear glasses or hearing aids? Who is your doctor? What kind of procedure are we doing today? Do you have any other health issues?"

After she checked over everything, it was time to take us into the pre-op holding area where they started Chris' IV. I looked away as the nurse inserted a needle into his vein and felt a little nauseous at the thought of it. I noticed the place was bustling with nurses and doctors getting patients ready for their procedures. Dr. Chehval came by to review and sign Chris' chart. He reminded us that the surgery should take about two hours and he would have someone notify me when they had started the procedure. He promised to see me in the waiting room afterwards.

"I'll meet you in the operating room, Chris," he said, shaking his hand. I realized that this was it and my heart began to race. I tried to get closer to Chris, but the bed rails were in the way. I reached in between the bars for his left hand, brought it to my lips, and kissed his fingers. He stroked my cheek with the back of his hand, smiling so sweetly that it made my knees quiver.

"No worries," he said.

Chris' anesthesiologist, Dr. Mary Faller, came and checked his IV. She took the time to get to know him through a list of standard questions and asking about his job, hobbies, and physical activities. When Chris introduced me, she congratulated us on our engagement. She was easy to talk to and had a great sense of humor. We connected with her right away. While she looked over Chris' chart, she sensed my nervousness and paused to assure me that Chris was in good hands with Dr. Chehval.

"He is one of the best surgeons around," she said.

"See, I told you that I have a really good feeling about him. It's all going to be okay, Steph," he said smiling. Dr. Faller walked back over to Chris' side and told us that it was time. She explained that once the "happy medicine" was given, they would need to take him into the operating room right away.

"Do you have any questions before we get started?" she asked the both of us.

"Nope, let's do it doc," Chris said and Dr. Faller injected the medicine into his IV.

"Give your pretty fiancée a kiss goodbye, Chris," she said. He looked at her with a boyish grin.

"What? It's not goodbye, it's 'I'll see you later,'" he said.

I laughed and leaned over the railing.

"I'll see you later," I whispered.

I stayed by Chris' side while Dr. Faller and a nurse pushed his bed out of the pre-op area. I felt a lump in my throat and squeezed his hand one more time.

"I'll be waiting for you," I choked.

"I... love... you...," he slurred, his eyes already droopy.

"We'll take good care of him," Dr. Faller promised and wheeled him away from me, down the hall, and through the doors into the operating room. *Oh God, please let everything go well.* When they disappeared, I felt sick to my stomach, standing there in the middle of the hallway. I couldn't move. *God, help me to be strong.* I don't know how long I stood there, but a staff member stopped and asked if I needed any help. I couldn't find my voice. She looked in the direction I was facing and seemed to understand what had just happened. She assured me that my loved one was in good hands and walked me back to the waiting area. Then I was left alone once again.

Feeling stranded, I looked around the crowded room for a friendly face, but everyone was preoccupied: some were reading, others were watching television, and a few of them were talking either on their cell phone or to someone next to them. *Why didn't I think to ask someone to sit with me?*

I bowed my head into my hands and talked to God. *Be with Chris, Dr. Chehval, Dr. Faller, and the nurses in that operating room. Give Dr. Chehval wisdom in his skill and expertise and guide his hands to remove the cancer from Chris' body. I ask you Lord for complete healing from this cancer and the strength Chris will need for recovery.* I kept repeating my prayer until I was strongly led to get my Bible. Turning the pages, I didn't know what I was looking for.

God, what do you want me to do? I flipped to the New Testament and ended up stopping at Matthew 11:28 – 30,

"Come to me, all you who work hard and who carry heavy burdens and I will refresh you. Take my yoke upon you and learn from me for I am gentle and humble of heart; and you will find rest. For my yoke is good and my burden is light."

I studied over the words, *"Come to me, who carry heavy burdens."* I realized my burdens were my worries and fear of this cancer that I was supposed to let go for God to take care of and He *"will refresh"* me. It was not an option to give up in the battle against this cancer, but I had to learn how to fight it effectively. By taking God's *"yoke"* meant that He would give me whatever I needed to be able to carry the load in our fight.

A yoke is a frame that joins two animals to do work, or it can rest on a person's shoulders to carry two equal loads, one on each end.

I was supposed to take God's yoke, but it wouldn't be heavy, it would be light – which is His grace and the kind of peace that is beyond my understanding, but I could feel it in my heart. To carry this load and to keep riding on in this race with Chris, I needed to get into God's Word to strengthen my faith.

I thought about the scripture and held onto my hope that Chris would be free from this cancer.

Before I knew it, I saw Chris' brothers, Mark and Patrick, rushing through the main entrance, looking around the waiting room frantically. I ran up to them.

"How's Chris?" they blurted.

"He's still in surgery, and he's doing well." Mark took a deep breath and Pat nodded. I wasn't used to seeing them so serious. They were always so easygoing and in a good mood. Mark was the one who offered encouragement and told stories that would make you laugh until your stomach hurt and Patrick took on the appearance of strength and power that made you feel safe and protected.

We waited together in silence until my cell phone rang. It was Teddie Momma and I had to step outside to get a better reception. She prayed for me to stay strong in my faith and for God's healing over Chris. And once again, I felt peace within me that was beyond my understanding.

Through the glass doors, I saw Dr. Chehval standing next to the information desk. I quickly said goodbye to Teddie, pushed through the door and ran into Mark.

"Stephanie, it's okay. Dr. Chehval just walked in." I took a deep breath and walked quickly over to Chris' doctor.

"Chris is in the recovery room and is doing well. I was able to remove the tumor and will send it over to the pathology lab for further tests and analysis. It will take several days before we get the results back. Depending upon how long it will take for Chris to wake up and recuperate from anesthesia, he'll be in the recovery room for another hour or so. Someone at the information desk will let you know his room number soon and he'll be admitted for several days. But right now, everything looks good."

Mark and Pat thanked Dr. Chehval and shook his hand. I hugged the man Chris trusted with his life.

"Thank you for taking care of him," I whispered.

"God, thank you!" I prayed, hugging Mark and Pat.

When we found out Chris' hospital room, we went there to wait for him. It seemed like days rather than hours had gone by since we last saw each other. I got busy checking out his room and unpacked his bag. Still, it felt like it was too long and Pat went to the nurses' station to find out what was happening when Mark saw Chris in the hospital bed coming down the hall. I stepped out to see him. After hearing my voice, he puckered his lips together as if he were kissing me. I leaned over the rail and met his lips.

After Chris was settled in his room, we walked in and he stretched his hand out to me, but I was limited in getting close to him by the guard rail. I was beginning to despise the barrier it created between us.

"How did it go?" he asked.

"Dr. Chehval removed the tumor and everything went well." He smiled, gave a thumb up with his free hand, and winked. He turned to his brothers.

"Hey man, how... you doing?" he asked.

I watched the three men reunite, talking as if they picked up where they left off from the last time they were together. Chris started perking up, following along with Mark and Pat while he drank apple juice and ate a few graham crackers. He was already looking like his old self again.

It wasn't long before we had to leave and it was the hardest thing I had to do. I wished I could stay and be with him.

"Goodnight babe. I'll talk to you first thing in the morning," I whispered.

"Goodnight," he yawned then leaned back into his pillow, already drifting to sleep. Mark put his arm around my shoulders.

"He'll be alright, Stephanie. He'll get a good night's sleep. Pat and I will spend the day with him tomorrow," he said.

I knew Mark was right and his comfort put me more at ease, but I still didn't like leaving Chris behind in the hospital, alone.

On the way home, I realized I was worrying again. When would I learn to let things go to God? Frustrated, I thought about the scripture from Matthew and asked myself what I was worried about. I didn't want to leave Chris alone. What if something goes wrong during the night? What if he needed me and I wasn't there by his side like I promised him? Each question added more weight – more burdens – in my chest. I couldn't do this to myself. Chris wouldn't want me to and neither would God. I needed to let go and trust Him to take care of my worries for me. I realized that I had a lot to learn about God's Word and to understand what He was trying to teach me.

I began to pray: *Okay God. I don't want to worry. So I'm going to believe nothing is going to go wrong because You will watch over Chris. We will both sleep peacefully and tomorrow will be the first day of healing for him. Thank You for bringing Mark and Pat here safely so they could be with Chris. A brother's love is a special bond you created that is so strong between them. I truly believe everything is going to be okay.* By the time I pulled in my garage, I felt a surreal sense of calmness in my heart and I knew God heard my prayer. For it says,

"Don't fret. Instead of worrying, pray. Let petitions and praises shape your worries into prayers, letting God know your concerns. Before you know it, a sense of God's wholeness, everything coming together for good, will come and settle you down. It's wonderful what happens when Christ displaces worry at the center of your life."

- Philippians 4:6 – 7

No one can handle anything better than God.

Just a Little Bump on the Road

"...hope does not disappoint."

- Romans 5:5

After four days in the hospital, Chris was released. He was already dressed when I arrived early that morning. A nurse gave us the supplies and reviewed the instructions on how to change his surgical bandages at home. Chris didn't pay much attention and finished packing his bag. I had never seen him so anxious. After she left, I tried to calm him down and he became agitated.

"Go get the car. I don't want to be here any longer than I have to," he snapped.

I knew it was better for the both of us to give him some space. When I pulled up to the entrance, someone was pushing Chris in a wheelchair up to the curb. Seeing his disgusted expression, I knew he wasn't pleased. The man barely stopped when Chris jumped out of it.

"I'm fine, you can go now," and uttered a barely audible "Thanks."

After I helped him get settled in the car, he leaned his head back.

"I'm sorry, Steph. I had had enough of being in the hospital and was starting to get stir-crazy." I couldn't blame him.

"Don't worry about it. You can relax now that we're on our way to your place."

"There is no place like home," Chris started saying and after the third time, he opened his eyes to see we were idling at a stop light.

"Sorry Chris, I don't have one of those magical hot-air balloons that would take you home in a blink of an eye," I said, laughing.

When Chris walked into the kitchen, I tried to keep D'Artagnon calm, but he was barking incessantly and trying to push his head into Chris' legs for him to rub his sides. It was hard to control a 90-pound excited Malamute.

"There really is no place like home," Chris said grinning wide, petting his dog.

Over the next couple of days, Chris struggled with the catheter and experienced a lot of pain from the surgical wounds. By late Monday afternoon, it bothered him so much that he called Dr. Chehval's office and was told to come in first thing the next day.

I went with Chris to his appointment and waited while Dr. Chehval met with him privately. Afterwards, Dr. Chehval asked me to come in so he could talk to the both of us. I felt a nervous twitch in my stomach, wondering what he was going to tell us.

"Are you feeling better," I asked.

"A little bit. Dr. Chehval cleaned the surgical wound and ordered a urinalysis to check for an infection. He replaced the catheter. I have to wear it for two more days and then hopefully he'll be able to remove it for good," he said somberly.

Dr. Chehval walked in holding Chris' file.

"How do you feel, Chris?" he asked.

"I'm starting to feel better. Thanks."

"I received the pathology results of the tumor I removed." He opened Chris' file. "It reported that 98 percent of the tumor has been removed," he paused and I held my breath. I stared at the doctor, trying to grasp what he was telling us.

"It was a challenge to remove the tumor since it was very close to the prostate and the sphincter muscle, which gives you the ability to contract or release to void." Dr. Chehval said. "I thought I got it all but wanted to be sure, which was why I sent it to the lab. I would like to consult with the team to brainstorm how to remove the rest of the tumor without interfering with the prostate and the sphincter muscle."

We were both quiet for the next several minutes.

"Okay," Chris said and shook Dr. Chehval's hand and thanked him again.

What does this mean? Is Chris in danger from having a part of the tumor still inside of him? What are we dealing with that is proving to be more difficult to fight against? My pulse started racing faster than the thoughts running through my mind and I was afraid of what this cancer was doing to Chris. I took several deep breaths to calm down. *God, this cancer scares me. What do we do next?* I opened my calendar book to write down Chris' appointment and saw a scripture from 2nd Timothy 1:7,

"God did not give us a spirit of fear, but of power, of love, and of a sound mind."

Feeling like I got a response, I calmed down. *Okay God, let's get some power over this thing.*

Chris was especially quiet when we walked out of the building. I tried to distract him, suggesting that we go somewhere, but he was anxious to get back home.

"I just want to work on my model and get my mind off of this for a while," he said.

Ever since Chris was a boy, he built models as a way to escape from life's difficulties. But now, it helped him find serenity and inner joy. Over the years, he continued to be fascinated with the history of war, tanks, and aircraft – especially the military planes. Chris developed a strong respect and admiration for the World War II fighter planes (those that were propeller-driven), the Korean War jets, and the Vietnam War fighter jets up to the modern day jets used in the Gulf War. His specialty in building these aircraft models were in using a foil method which can be very challenging – a wrong cut or placement of the foil could cause a permanent error, ruining the model. He was extremely meticulous in his attention to every detail with his skills in painting, especially of the cockpits in the planes and the tiny figurines. These two skills required a lot of patience and effort which Chris improved upon by working on many different models and by using various techniques and strategies he learned through magazines, workshops, club meetings, and networking with others.

Chris' passion for his hobby grew and he accumulated anything and everything he needed and wanted to build models and create dioramas: paint, decals, brushes, tools, light settings, magnifying glasses, books and magazines, photographs and posters, a variety of landscapes, buildings, planes, vehicles, and GI Joe's. He collected a variety of kits, feeling the freedom to have as many as he wanted without anyone telling him otherwise. Chris' work was recognized and admired in open displays and contests from which he earned many awards and trophies. Whenever people complimented him, Chris would be humble and very gracious, but he would find ways to improve his skills. To share his love of the hobby, he joined two clubs: the International Plastic Models Society (IPMS) and Mastercon. In the IPMS of St. Louis, Chris served as the club's President, Vice-President, Secretary, Treasurer, and Vendor Organizer. Other vendors, colleagues, friends, and customers gravitated toward him because of his enthusiasm, leadership, and talents for the craft.

Chris loved building models so much that he'd find ways to share it with others and was often generous with them. As his way of honoring the United States Veterans of all wars, he donated several pieces of his work to a museum in downtown St. Louis. Sometimes, he'd feel a strong intuition to build a particular model for someone and he'd stop whatever project he was on until it was completed.

One of my favorite projects was a diorama of a 1993 Missouri flood scene showing the Coast Guard rescuing a person and his dog on top of a roof as a dedication to his brother, Patrick.

After meeting Grandpa Schoonover, Chris built a model of the USS Stevens, the destroyer Grandpa served on during World War II.

Another time, Chris spent hours researching for a model on the type of helicopter my brother, Rich, was currently flying and built it for him.

Even though I didn't like Chris being alone so much, I knew he needed to escape and to process things in his own way. Working on a model gives him the time to do this.

I realized that I needed some time to myself too. I had been so busy with my job, taking care of my dogs and my house, and planning our wedding while being there for Chris that I was exhausted. I had no idea I was dealing with so much at once and the winter break from school came at just the right time.

After a couple of days of catching up on things, I was free to be with Chris and was so happy to see him in better spirits.

"Steph, I feel like I have a better handle on getting through my recovery. I just need to take it one day at a time and not think about tomorrow so much. But no matter what happens next, I am not going to give up. There is always hope. God will give me the strength to keep on fighting."

Chris wanted to see Dr. Chehval on his own and promised to let me know what happened. I hoped and prayed Chris would be relieved from the catheter. For an early morning appointment, it wasn't until several hours later when he finally called me.

"Chris, are you okay?" I blurted.

"Hey Babe, I'm great," he said cheerfully. "The catheter is out and I'm doing well without it. I have a follow-up appointment with Dr. Chehval next Thursday and he hopes to know more on what to do about the rest of the tumor. It's all good, Steph."

Oh thank you, God. We needed some good news and I continued to pray for healing in Chris' body.

Even though Chris didn't have to deal with the catheter anymore, he was still miserable and agitated from the surgical wounds. It was hard for me to understand what he was going through, not being able to see what had been done to him and I tried to be patient. I hoped he'd feel better by Christmas day.

"Spend time with your family, Steph. We'll do Christmas together later." I knew he'd be more at ease at home but it wasn't supposed to be like this. I didn't like the idea of him being alone part of the day and the burden of it was heavy in my heart. Sensing my hesitation on the phone, he continued, "This is the best I can do, Steph. It's too uncomfortable for me to move around and I'm always going to the bathroom. It would be better for me to stay home. I'll stay busy with one of my models and the hours will go by fast, and then you'll be here."

"Okay, Chris," I said reluctantly. "But if you need anything, please call me," and he promised he would.

I tried to enjoy Christmas at my sister's house. It was fun watching my nieces, nephews, and great-nephews open their gifts excitedly and seeing the awe on their faces when Santa came by for a quick visit. Chris would have loved this and I felt the cancer was cheating us out of what would have been a wonderful day for us.

The weight of the despair I felt all afternoon was finally released the moment I was in Chris' arms.

"I know this hasn't been an easy day. I'm proud of you for being so strong for your family and for me. But I want you to know something, Steph," and he tilted my chin to face him and pointed to my heart, "no matter what happens – if we can't be together – we will never be apart."

I nodded and held him tightly, not wanting to let him go.

"But right now we are together and I don't want to think about us being apart."

I spent most of my time off with Chris. We watched movies and played board games, but we had to pause a lot so he could go to the bathroom. I prayed and hoped this was a good sign that his body was healing.

Before we knew it, we were back with Dr. Chehval for Chris' follow-up. After he examined Chris, I was called from the waiting room to meet them in Dr. Chehval's office. I didn't like the idea of returning to his office and fought my nervousness. I sat in the chair next to Chris and he held my hand.

"Chris is healing nicely. It's just going to take some time," Dr. Chehval told me. "I've been doing some research and talked with a team of specialists here. We need to figure out a way to get the rest of the tumor out without interfering with the sphincter muscle. If you want to go ahead with another surgery, Chris, then we would need to assess the margins of the tumor and its distance from the sphincter muscle."

"Let's do it, doctor," Chris said determined to get back into the fight. The test was scheduled during the second week of January, about a week-and-a-half-away. I didn't like having to wait another two weeks to find out the results. Chris squeezed my hand, bringing me out of my thoughts.

"Don't worry, Steph. We have a lot to look forward to, 2006 is going to be our year. We'll beat this cancer and I'll get back on my bike. We'll have many more happy moments, especially our wedding day and," he paused, kissing the side of my neck, "our honeymoon. I have a lot to live for."

I knew God would continue to be there for us and help us in our race to victory at the finish line. For it says in Romans 12:12,

"Have hope and be cheerful. Be patient in trials and pray constantly."

To my surprise, the days passed by quickly ringing in the New Year and starting a new semester. Before I knew it, it was time to meet with Dr. Chehval to find out the results of the test. We sat together at a small round table in his office.

"The tumor is very close to the sphincter muscle at exactly 1.2 cm from it. It would be difficult to remove it without interfering with Chris' ability to control urinary functions," Dr. Chehval explained, showing us on the model. "There is a specialist who has had some experience in this kind of surgery and I recommend for you to see him and hear his opinion on what to do."

"Okay, let's set it up," Chris said.

Later on that day, Chris called excited that the meeting with the new doctor was scheduled for the following Thursday. I was thrilled that we didn't have to wait so long. I felt like we were moving in the right direction.

Over the weekend, we had dinner with Bob, Kelly, and their children, and Chris shared the latest news with them.

"This is just a little bump on the road. You'll ride on over it, Chris," Bob said confidently.

"And we'll keep praying for you," Kelly said.

There was so much hope around us at that moment I felt goose bumps all over my arms and legs. I was speechless. I continued to be amazed at how God works through others for us. For it says,

"...hope does not disappoint, because [of] *the love of God."*
- Romans 5:5

Dead End

"Let us hold fast to our hope without wavering, because He who promised is faithful."

- Hebrews 10:23

Chris and I couldn't wait to meet this new doctor and I wondered what he was like. The building we walked into was twice the size as the cancer center we were used to. The waiting room was decorated in deep shades of mahogany, hunter green and maroon colors giving the sense of luxury for a medical building.

When a receptionist called Chris' name, we were taken into one of the patient rooms and were told that Dr. Croft would be in shortly. It felt like a moment of déjà-vu, one that seemed so familiar, but I knew it hadn't happened – yet. I started taking some deep breaths to shake this eerie feeling when the door suddenly opened and a short, stocky man with red curly hair walked in.

"Hello, I'm Dr. Croft," he said and shook Chris' hand.

"So, what brings you here?" he asked, leaning against the examining table and folding his arms across his chest.

What?! Doesn't he know why we are here?

Chris told him that he was recommended by Dr. Chehval for a second opinion about the tumor in the urethra

"That's a rare type of cancer," he said, glancing at me and then at Chris. "Okay, start at the beginning and tell me everything you've done so far." He sat down on a stool, opened Chris' thin file and started taking notes while Chris summarized the details from the discovery of the lump to the surgery. After a series of questions, Dr. Croft admitted that he had not seen any of Chris' records, but he would call his assistant to look into it.

"I'm unable to give you my opinion until I look over your scans and reports. We will need to reschedule. I suggest you call Dr. Chehval's office and ask them to forward your records to me as soon as possible."

We found out that it would be two weeks until we could see Dr. Croft again.

"That's the earliest date we can get?" I asked the receptionist. She offered to call us if there was a cancellation. Dumbfounded, my hands shook, writing the appointment down in my calendar. When we got back into Chris' SUV, he let off some steam.

"I can't believe he didn't know why I was there! Didn't he get my records? I know Dr. Chehval's office sent them over. Now I have to wait two more weeks while this thing is inside of me. I just want to get it out!" He slammed the steering wheel with his fist. "How can I fight this when I have to keep waiting for the doctors to figure out what to do?"

I didn't know what I could say that would make this better for him. I just listened to him vent. When he was out of breath, he put the car in gear and drove us away.

"I can't believe I have to come back here," he mumbled.

I shook my head, feeling the same way. I really thought we were on our way in this fight, but we hadn't gotten anywhere. It felt like we reached a dead-end. Where do we go from here?

When Chris parked the car in his garage, he turned off the ignition, and sat there.

"I'm sorry for going off like that. Thanks for being here for me."

"Chris, I know you're disappointed about today and I am too. I feel your anger and frustration. I want you to know that it's okay to let it out and I'll listen."

We talked about Dr. Croft. Chris wasn't sure if he liked him, but he knew this doctor was supposed to be one of the best. We couldn't understand how he didn't have a copy of Chris' record and Chris planned to call Dr. Chehval's office first thing in the morning to work it out.

I wondered how we would get through the next 14 days before we would know which direction to go. Chris and I realized that we needed to stay faithful in our hope for healing, trust God that He was in control, and continue to pray.

"May God, the source of hope, fill you with joy and peace in the faith so that your hope may increase by the power of the Holy Spirit."
- Romans 15:13

We took each day one at a time. Chris was finally released to return to work in the Gaming Division at one of the casinos and completed a weekend drill for the Air National Guard. Even though he was doing things again, he was still dealing with the physical challenges of his body healing from the surgery. One day, Chris had to leave work suddenly because he wasn't able to urinate. Dr. Chehval relieved the scar tissue that caused the blockage and re-inserted a catheter for Chris to wear 24 hours, forcing him to take another sick day.

Since we were able to stay busy, it hadn't been so hard waiting to meet with Dr. Croft again, but it was long enough.

After briefly reviewing Chris' thicker file, he closed it shut and put it on the desk.

"Yours is not a simple case," he said matter-of-factly. "There are a couple of options we can look at: the first is to remove the urethra and reconstruct it with a skin graft, however there is a risk of the cancer returning. The second option, and I strongly recommend this, is to remove part of the urethra, the external sphincter muscle, part of the prostate, and the bladder. The more aggressive we are to treat this cancer, the better the chances are for your survival."

I stared at the doctor. I couldn't swallow or find my voice to speak.

"Doc...," Chris cleared his throat, "Dr. Croft, how would I be able to relieve myself?"

"I would create an incision just below your belly button and insert a tube with a balloon to where your bladder used to be which means you will wear a catheter with a bag." I clenched my jaws together so tightly that I started to feel the pain behind my ears and a headache began to form.

Oh my God, what does this mean for Chris' quality of life? He is only 47-years-old.

Chris cleared his throat again and leaned forward, resting his elbows on his knees.

"Doctor, I'm a physically active person. It's a part of who I am – an athlete. I ride my bicycle and compete in races. I run and I play with my dog. I'm a police officer and I work as a weapons technician on the fighter jets in the Air National Guard. Steph and I are getting married in June and we plan to have a family. I want to help take care of my children and play with them someday. How am I supposed to do all of that wearing a bag?"

I finally looked at Chris and saw tears in his eyes. *Lord, give us the strength we need right now, this is too much.*

"I understand," Dr. Croft nodded.

Startled, I wanted to tell this doctor that he couldn't possibly understand – that he didn't get who Chris was and what he was trying to tell him.

"But we have to take aggressive measures. You have a rare cancer for which there is no common consensus on treatment. We are talking about doing whatever it takes to save your life," Dr. Croft said.

Death? Oh God, please help us. We're both barely hanging on.

"What about trying other kinds of chemotherapy?" Chris asked.

"I'm afraid that would be a waste of time. You tried Cisplatin, which is a very strong drug that should have made a difference to the tumor, but it grew nonetheless. Chemotherapy didn't cure it."

"Okay, what about radiation?" Chris asked, still not giving up. Dr. Croft shook his head, pressing his lips together looking frustrated.

"Again, I'm sorry but since chemo didn't work, the chances of radiation being effective are very slim and it would cause terrible pain for you."

Oh my God. I struggled to breathe, feeling the weight of all of this building up in my chest, but Chris still hung on to his hope.

"Could we try laser surgery on the tumor?"

"That may work to keep the tumor from growing further and your body could dispose it, however there is a very strong chance that another tumor would develop and nothing would be solved. You would find yourself back here again. You have a very complicated case. There are no simple solutions, which is why we need to take drastic measures."

I wanted the doctor to stop talking. It felt like I was going from one shock to another. It was too much. *Could this really be happening? If this is a bad dream, wake up. WAKE UP!*

I closed my eyes and opened them to find Chris rubbing his jaw. There was an awkward silence in the room that made me shiver.

"Do you have any more questions?" Dr. Croft asked.

"No, I can't think of any. Steph?" Our eyes met for the first time. He was still fighting for composure and I struggled to swallow the lump in my throat. "Do you have anything you want to ask?" Still unable to find my voice, I shook my head.

"I'll send my report to Dr. Chehval and you can discuss it together before making a decision." He stood up and shook Chris' hand, "Good luck," and the doctor quickly walked out of the door. I put our binder in my backpack and picked up my purse.

"Let's get out of here," Chris said angrily, grabbing my hand.

I couldn't stop my body from shaking. I continued to fight the tears as my headache grew more intense.

"I want to go over to the infertility clinic. I need to make sure everything is secure to still be able to have our family," Chris said. There was a sense of urgency about him, walking briskly across the campus to the building where the office was located. I had a hard time keeping up with his long strides.

When we found out that everything was okay, Chris calmed down and took a deep breath.

"Good," he whispered.

But I was still trying to wrap my head around our meeting with Dr. Croft. Once in the car, I couldn't hold it in any more – the weight in my chest, the lump growing in my throat, and the headache that was throbbing against my forehead – I lost it.

"I'm sorry," I cried. "I am so sorry. I should be strong for you and the last thing you need is to see me like this. I love you so much and I hate that this is happening to you. I wish I could do something to take this all away from you and make things better."

"I know, Steph. I don't like seeing you cry, but I know it's because you love me and you care so much," he said and kissed my hand.

I kept taking deep breaths to calm down while Chris drove. Every time I thought about what Dr. Croft told us, I'd feel the weight of its heavy burden in my chest again.

"Chris, drive to Dr. Chehval's office."

"We don't have an appointment with him," he said.

"I don't care. I need to see him. *Now*. I am not going to wait another week or even another day to talk to him about Dr. Croft's opinion. I'll wait there all afternoon if I have to, but I will see him today."

Chris had never seen me like this and called Dr. Chehval's office.

"They said to come on in," he said, smiling. I watched Chris exit off the highway and noticed how composed he had been since we left.

"How can you be so calm?" I yelled. "After hearing such horrifying news, I can't stop crying. How do you do it, Chris?"

I will always remember exactly how he responded and the serene expression he showed when he answered me.

"Steph, I take a deep breath, hold it, then let it out and as I do, I lift my hands up to God and pray, 'God, take this. You can deal with it much better than I can. I don't know what to do, but You do. I am not going to worry about this. I've got to stay focused on my fight here. So, I'm letting it go to You. Thank you.' I stay quiet for a few minutes and then I'd feel peace in my heart. I'm okay. I can keep fighting."

Chris knew how to put his faith in God in moments like these and he wasn't at a dead-end. I still needed to learn how to turn to God first, rather than let fear or my emotions overwhelm me.

"Cast your burden on the Lord and He will sustain you; He will never let the righteous fall."

- Psalm 55:22

Watching Chris at that moment, he looked so strong and confident. Chris' faith made him hopeful and peaceful. It reminded me of the scripture from Second Timothy 1:7,

"God has not given me the spirit of fear, but of power, love, and a sound mind."

Because Chris continued to give up troubling things to God, I truly believed God blessed him to keep riding on strong in his race.

When we walked into Dr. Chehval's office, Sarah, one of the nurses on his staff, took us into his private office and told us that he would be in soon. Before leaving, she paused and squeezed my shoulder empathetically. I took several deep breaths to stay in control.

"Steph," Chris whispered, "it's going to be okay." He stroked my cheek with his thumb and held my hand. The door opened and Dr. Chehval walked into the room and sat at the table with us.

"Doctor, I appreciate taking the time from your busy schedule to see us. We just saw Dr. Croft and we needed to talk to you about his opinion." He nodded and folded his hands on the table, listening intensely while Chris told him about our meeting. Once again, I was amazed at his composure while he shared the specific details.

"Dr. Chehval," I interrupted, "you know Chris and how physically active he is. How can he have a good quality of life with a bag at his side? How is he to ride his bike, play with his dog," I choked, "and play with our children someday?"

"I know it was very difficult to hear Dr. Croft's opinion," Dr. Chehval said. "He is an expert, which is why I wanted you to see him. After I look over his notes, we'll meet again to discuss your options and go from there. Okay?"

Chris looked at me and I nodded. But what I really wanted was for Dr. Chehval to disagree with Dr. Croft and give us renewed hope to find a better solution for Chris.

"Thank you for your time," Chris said and shook his doctor's hand.

When we left, my head was pounding so hard, I was beginning to feel nauseous. I had had enough for the day.

"Are you feeling better?" Chris asked.

"Yes," I sighed, not wanting to tell him how I really felt. "I'm glad we talked to Dr. Chehval. You have strong instincts, Chris. Dr. Chehval is a very good doctor for you."

"Well of course I have good instincts," he said, pulling me close to him. "I chose you to spend the rest of my life with, didn't I?" he asked, tickling my neck with his lips, making me laugh.

We had no idea how long it would be before hearing from Dr. Chehval, so we stayed busy with our jobs, our dogs, our homes, and continued planning our wedding. I was also getting my house ready to put on the market.

On Valentine's Day, Chris had problems voiding and began to feel the pressure in his bladder. He went in to see Dr. Chehval, but he was on vacation. So Chris saw Dr. Hoffman, who took his call. He was able to clear the scar tissue out of the way. Chris had to wear a catheter again for a couple of days and then he was able to void on his own.

However, two weeks later, he had the same problems again. This was the third time within six weeks. Dr. Chehval wanted to do a cystoscopy so he could remove the scar tissue and reinsert the catheter. Chris didn't care. He would do anything to prevent it from building up again. He called me at school, needing me to be there for him. My school secretary managed to get a sub for me quickly and I hurried over to the surgery center. By the time I got there, Chris was already in the pre-op area. Dr. Faller was his anesthesiologist and we were happy to see her again. She reminded me that Chris was in good hands and I watched her take him into the operating room.

Feeling alone, I took a deep breath and let it out slowly. I returned to the waiting room trying to figure out how to fill this emptiness. I remembered what Chris told me that day after seeing Dr. Croft. I closed my eyes and imagined raising my hands up to God.

Okay, Lord. I don't want to feel this way and I'm giving it to you. I will not be afraid and I am not going to worry. Guide Dr. Chehval in the operating room and show him what to do for Chris. I know You are taking care of Chris and helping us stay strong together. Thank you for blessing us with a special love.

I was so focused in my prayer that I didn't realize Dr. Chehval called my name until he sat next to me. I nearly jumped when I felt his hand on my shoulder.

"Is everything okay?" I asked, startled.

"Everything is fine," he said. "I was able to remove the scar tissue easily and Chris is recovering well. He will have to wear the catheter for 24 hours. He can come by my office tomorrow afternoon to have it removed," he said. Then he noticed the Bible on my lap.

"Is that your Bible?"

"I've been praying and reading over some scriptures," I told him.

He took my hand with both of his hands.

"Do me a favor," he paused and looked in my eyes, "pray for me, too?" he asked.

"Oh, Dr. Chehval, I have been," I exclaimed and he smiled. He squeezed my hand and placed it back on my Bible.

"Thank you." he whispered. "Someone will call you soon when Chris is in a room and you can be with him again."

I watched him walk away and thanked God for bringing Dr. Chehval into our lives and for taking good care of Chris.

After a while, I took Chris home and spoiled him the rest of the day. He did well recuperating from the procedure and tolerated the catheter. The next day, Chris was able to void on his own. He called me after school to tell me the good news.

"Dr. Chehval received Dr. Croft's notes and he wants to meet with the team to review it. I have a PET scan scheduled at the beginning of March and then we'll meet with him the following week to find out our next step. It's all good, Steph. I feel like we're finding our way back into the fight again."

I hope so. Lead us in the right direction, Oh Lord.

It felt like the longest two weeks, waiting to know what Dr. Chehval would tell us. *What if he agreed with Dr.* Croft's *opinion? Chris trusts Dr. Chehval, so how would he handle this kind of news? How could I help him through this?* These questions swirled around in my mind, making me more nervous. I realized what I was doing to myself and decided to turn all my worries over to God. It was beyond what I could handle and I prayed to Him for strength and patience.

"I can do all things in Christ Jesus who strengthens me."
- Philippians 4:13

While we waited for Dr. Chehval in his office, I kept fidgeting with my pen and jiggling my knee. I caught Chris' eye and stopped.

"Steph," Chris whispered, "it's going to be okay."

Dr. Chehval walked in, asked Chris how he was feeling, and then shook my hand. After he sat down at his desk, he began to tell us the results of the test.

"The PET scan showed the one tumor that is left in the urethra," he said.

This is very good news. Thank you, God.

"After reviewing Dr. Croft's notes and discussing them with the team here, it would be best to remove the rest of the tumor, the sphincter muscle, and a small part of the prostate. I do not think it's necessary to remove the bladder, but we would need to look inside it to make sure it is clear of the cancer and healthy."

Chris let go of my hand, leaned forward with his elbows on his knees and rested his chin on his hands. He pressed his lips tightly and pulled his eyebrows together in deep thought.

"Is there any way we could save the sphincter muscle since it's important for urinary control?" I asked.

"Because of the close proximity of the tumor next to it, there is a strong chance of interfering with the muscle while removing the rest of the tumor," Dr. Chehval explained. "Since the prostate is within the area, I would have to remove a small portion that is closest to it."

No matter what our options were or what Chris decided to do, some of his body would have to be sacrificed. *What kind of changes would he need to adjust to? How would this affect his feelings as a man?*

"Chris, there is no other way around it. Unfortunately, we will need to take these aggressive measures to remove the tumor," Dr. Chehval said.

"Let's do it," Chris piped up suddenly.

"Okay. If you want Dr. Croft to do the surgery, I can..." Chris interrupted.

"No, I don't trust anyone else to operate on me but you Doctor – that is if you are comfortable doing this surgery?"

"I can do it, Chris," he said. We found out the surgery was scheduled in six days. I took a deep breath and thanked God we didn't have to wait very long again.

"We're back in the fight, Steph," he said, smiling confidently. It felt like we had found our way out of the dead-end and we were riding on again.

"*So let's do it – full of belief. Let's keep a firm grip on the promises that keep us going. He always keeps His word. Let's see how inventive we can be in encouraging love.*"

- Hebrews 10:22, 23

Strength and Blessings

"The Lord will give strength to His people. The Lord will bless His people with peace."

- Psalm 29:11

One night over the weekend, Teddie Momma and her husband, Dan – who we called Fitz – came over to my house to have dinner with us.

"You have a special story to tell," Fitz told us. "You have been blessed with an amazing love for each other that many today dream and hope to find. You were meant to fight the good fight of faith. You've already gone through some tough battles and yet, you grow stronger in your faith and hope, believing God will take care of you.

The Bible tells us that we would suffer trials, persecutions, and tests. Those who persevered in their faith will have victory in Jesus and become a witness for others. Teddie and I believe God brought you together to endure this race and Jesus will bring you to victory because you will have a strong testimony to share with others." He quoted 2nd Corinthians 2:14,

"Thanks be to God, who always lead us in victory through Christ Jesus and, through us, spreads the knowledge of Him everywhere."

"Chris, you've been through a lot already and you continued to carry on in your race. Stay strong in believing for your healing." Then Fitz turned to me and continued, "Stephanie, no matter what news you hear, trust God, who is in control of everything." He reached across the table and held our hands. "Through all of this, Chris and Stephanie, let your love grow so deep that it will shine and be a light for others."

"In Christ Jesus, the only thing that counts is faith expressing itself through love."

- Galatians 5:6

After they left, Chris and I talked about what Fitz told us. We realized that we needed to include our families and friends on what was going on while sharing our faith and hope with them. So, I started an e-mail group with everyone I could think of to give them updates and to join us in praying for Chris' healing.

"For where two or three come together in My Name, there I am with them."

- Matthew 18:20

With the surgery just days away, I knew I couldn't wait by myself again and asked those closest to us if anyone was available to sit with me. Teddie, Bob, and his parents, Momma Sue and Poppa Bob, responded eagerly and I knew I would be in good hands.

As Chris was getting prepped for surgery, a nurse overheard us talking about our friends being there for us and she told us that we could have one additional visitor. Knowing just who to get, I hurriedly rushed into the waiting room. When we rounded the corner to the other side of the curtain, I let Bob go ahead of me. He slowly made his way over to Chris with so much love and admiration in his eyes, I had to look away to brace myself. There was also a surge of energy about him and I could tell it affected Chris when he suddenly sat up straight and shook Bob's hand. They talked and joked together until Dr. Faller came and told us they were ready for him. Bob gave Chris a gentle shoulder hug, "See you later, good buddy."

"Ride on," Chris replied.

Dr. Faller already had given Chris the medicine and told him to give me a kiss. I leaned over the bed railing and he swerved to the right, grinning.

"Okay babe, let's try again." Before I knew it, Chris turned his face to the left, smiling coyly and winked at me with both eyes.

"It looks like the medicine is already working so we need to get Chris into the operating room," Dr. Faller said. I held his face in my hands.

"Third time's a charm," I said and he tried to swerve again, but I was able to get a quick kiss.

"Hmmm," he mumbled, moving his eyebrows up and down.

"All right, Chris, it's time to head out," Dr. Faller laughed. Chris suddenly sat up with his arms propped out in front of him, giving the impression he was driving and I noticed his right foot pressed down on the gurney as if he was stepping on a gas pedal.

"Move out," he shouted.

"Okay, Chris, but don't give me a ticket for my driving skills." Dr. Faller said.

"A ticket? Why would I give you a ticket?" Chris questioned. "You can't drive while you're intoxicated. Let's go," he yelled and pretended to honk his horn. I watched them disappear into the operating room and heard Chris yell, "Woo-hoo."

Standing there alone in the hallway, I felt another déjà-vu moment. I shook it off and hurried back to my friends.

"Bob, you're going to love this one," and told him about Chris.

"What a goofball," he said. "But I'm not surprised." It was good to laugh, especially during this time of waiting when it would have been intense for me had I been by myself. Bob had to go to work and we promised to keep him posted.

Two hours later, I saw Dr. Chehval step into the waiting room. I introduced him to everyone and he led me into a small room. I held my breath hoping everything was okay.

"Chris is doing fine," he started and I exhaled the tension from my lungs. "The surgery took longer than I expected. It was challenging to remove the tumor, but I think I got it all. I was able to save the sphincter muscle and took a very small part of the prostate, about the size of a button. I looked inside the bladder and did not see any signs of cancer. However, Chris lost a unit of blood during the operation and had to have a blood transfusion, but he is recovering well. He'll feel weak for a few days and will need a lot of rest. Overall, things look good."

"Thank you so much Dr. Chehval," I said, hugging him.

"I'll come by to see Chris later on," he promised.

Oh God, thank you. Thank you for working through Dr. Chehval.

I took another deep breath and walked slowly back into the waiting room like I was in a daze. Poppa came up to me, held my arm and helped me into the chair between Momma Sue and Teddie. They held my hands and Poppa knelt down before me, waiting to hear the news.

"Chris is cancer-free," I cried out. "I can't wait to tell him." We hugged and Teddie said a prayer of thanksgiving to God with us.

"It is good to give thanks to the Lord and to sing praises to His Name; for He is good, for His love endures forever. He sent forth His Word and healed them."

- Psalm 92:1 and 107:1, 20

I looked at my friends smiling at me and felt their love. Chris and I were blessed with so much more than each other. We had close family and good friends who would stand by our side through the happiest and hardest times of our lives. They stayed with me until they had to leave. But I wasn't alone very long when Mark showed up and I told him the news.

"Oh, that's great, great news, Stephanie," Mark said. He wiped his eyes and got on his cell phone to tell their brothers and his family. It was a little while longer when we were finally given Chris' room number. After sitting all afternoon, I was happy to move around.

"Steph, Chris is coming," Mark said from the hallway and I rushed out to see him. He was half awake, but alert enough to stretch his hand out to me.

"Hi," he said weakly.

"Hi Chris," I said and squeezed his hand. The nurse checked over him carefully and re-adjusted the IV bags of fluids and pain medicine. I stayed by his side and Mark stood at the foot of the bed. Chris finally noticed him when he looked up.

"Hey man...good to see you," Chris slurred.

"I'm glad to be here. How are you feeling?" he asked. Chris gave one thumb up and then turned to me with questioning eyes.

"Dr. Chehval thinks he got it all out."

"Good," he said, smiling and fell asleep. Mark and I stayed with Chris until I started feeling the effects from a very long day. I hated leaving him in the hospital, but it made it a little easier knowing Mark was there.

Driving home, I went through the day.

"Chris is cancer free," I cried out in my car. "God, thank you for guiding Dr. Chehval through the surgery and for taking good care of Chris." I continued to pray for Chris' healing and recovery from this surgery.

"Rejoice always, pray without ceasing, and give thanks to God at every moment. This is the will of God for you."
- 1st Thessalonians 5:16–18

I called Chris first thing the next morning and Dr. Chehval had already visited him. "The cancer is gone, Steph," he said excitedly.

"Thank God," I laughed and told him I would see him after school.

By the time I got to the hospital, Chris was in an irritable mood and I found out he had a difficult day dealing with the surgical wounds and the catheter. It wasn't long before Dr. Chehval walked in. Mark and I left so he could examine Chris. While we waited, I felt an overwhelming weight build in my chest and burst into tears. I didn't know what came over me and I felt a pair of strong arms pull me into a teddy bear hug.

"Steph, it's okay," Mark said. "Chris had a tough day, but he'll pull through. He's just agitated being in the hospital, but he's okay." I nodded, took several deep breaths to calm down. Mark started telling me some funny stories, making me laugh.

Dr. Chehval poked his head out and motioned for us to come back in. I made my way to Chris' side. He smiled weakly, resting his head on the pillows, and held my hand.

"The surgical wounds look good," Dr. Chehval told us. "I'll come by in the morning again to check on you, Chris. If you're doing better, you may be able to go home later in the afternoon."

"Good," Chris perked up.

"The most important thing to do right now is to rest which I think you could do much better at home than here."

"I'll do whatever you want me to do, Doctor, just as long I don't have to stay here any longer," Chris said. I followed Dr. Chehval into the hallway.

"Chris is okay Stephanie, but he's getting stressed being here. Since he lost a lot of blood, he's going to be weak for a few days. He needs a lot of rest to recuperate."

"I'll make sure he doesn't do anything he's not supposed to do," I promised.

When I walked back into the room, Chris was joking with Mark, already in a better mood. I could see the weariness in his eyes and I realized that he had a long way to go before he would get his strength back.

Soon after he ate some of his dinner, he fell asleep.

"Sleep well tonight, Chris. I'll call you in the morning," I whispered and kissed him on his forehead.

"Don't worry, Steph," Mark said. "I'll stay with him a little longer, but I'm sure he'll sleep through the night."

"I'm really glad you're here, Mark. Thank you for coming."

Walking out of the hospital, another wave of tears threatened. Chris endured so much of the fight physically while I dealt with it emotionally. I prayed for the kind of strength we each needed to keep riding on together.

The next day, Chris was already settled at home by the time school let out. Mark stayed through the weekend and helped Chris get around, prepared meals for him, and made sure he rested. Even though they already had a good relationship, I think they grew closer during this time they spent together. When Mark left early that Sunday, Chris stood in the driveway and watched his older brother drive down the street.

"Do you know who my heroes are, Steph?" he asked, wiping his eyes. "My brothers," he said proudly.

Throughout the week, Chris continued to recover from the surgery, but he had a hard time with the catheter. By Friday, he was in so much pain with it, he saw Dr. Chehval late that afternoon. He took the catheter out and waited for a while to make sure Chris was able to show self-control and void on his own, which he did without any difficulties. This was a good sign and Dr. Chehval gave Chris the rest of the night without the catheter, but wanted him to return to the office first thing Saturday morning so he could examine him again.

"Steph, everything is looking good and I don't have the catheter anymore." he said, excited.

Things were going in the right direction, and we were enjoying every moment.

Unseen Hope

"Faith is the way of holding onto what we hope for, being certain of what we cannot see."

- Hebrews 11:1

The week before Easter, I sold my house sooner than we expected. Even though a huge weight had been lifted, Chris and I agreed not to live together until our wedding day, which meant I didn't know where I would stay until then. Fortunately I was able to stay with one of my girlfriends for the next two months who lived ten minutes away from Chris, which allowed us to spend a little more time together.

One day, Chris asked me to take an afternoon off to go with him to a follow-up appointment with Dr. Chehval.

"Chris, your body is healing well from the surgery," Dr. Chehval said. "I've been staying in contact with Dr. Needles about your progress and he wants to order a PET scan." I felt a twinge of nervousness in the pit of my stomach. Sensing my tension, he continued. "This is to be proactive and to stay on top of things."

"I'm not worried, let's do it," Chris said confidently. I took a deep breath and looked at my fiancé who knew God was in control. He continued to inspire me to look deeper in my own faith.

"Blessed is the man who trusts in the Lord, whose confidence is in Him!"

- Jeremiah 17:7

Two weeks later, we learned there was no cancer activity in Chris' body. The test reported inconclusive below the pelvic area and was speculated to be scar tissue.

This was confirmed when Chris started having problems at the end of April, which was about five weeks after the surgery. Dr. Chehval helped Chris get some relief, but in order to clear the scar tissue and dilate the passageway completely, Chris would have to be put under mild anesthetics. It would be too painful for him to endure while conscious. Dr. Chehval scheduled the procedure for the end of the week.

By Saturday morning, as I drove Chris to the surgery center, he was beginning to feel the pressure build up in his bladder. Since it was a weekend, he was taken care of right away. Dr. Chehval told us the procedure would take about 20 minutes.

I walked back to the deserted waiting room. Waiting became an enemy, especially when I was by myself. I watched the blooming trees gently sway in the breeze and began to rock along with them, feeling the comfort of the branches as if they were God's arms wrapping around me, loving me and reminding me that He is our hope and would always be there for us.

"But this, when I ponder, is what gives me hope: because of the Lord's great love, we are not consumed. His compassions are new every morning. And His love remains ever faithful."

- Lamentations 3:21–23

I didn't have to wait very long when Dr. Chehval came out and sat next to me.

"It was scar tissue blocking the area preventing the urine from passing through. Now that Chris is dilated, he should feel much better."

When I met up with Chris, he was eating a graham cracker.

"What's up, babe?" he asked smiling. I couldn't help but laugh, feeling relieved to see Chris doing well.

Over the next week, Chris and I worked together to rearrange our house with both of our things, getting more excited to live together soon. But he continued to have problems and had to be dilated two more times. He never complained and if he was frustrated, he didn't show it. Chris trusted God that He was in control over everything. He stayed focused on what he had to do to get better. He lived one day at a time and stayed strong in his will to keep riding on.

When Chris and I entered the surgery center the fourth time in May for the dilation procedure, we knew the routine and had gotten to know the staff better. We'd grown fond of Chris' anesthesiologist, Dr. Faller, who always shared our sense of humor. And whenever Dr. Chehval came by to sign off Chris' chart, the pre-op room would be on a roll with jibes and jokes.

Everything went as well as expected, but when Dr. Chehval talked to me, he mentioned doing a biopsy. Even though I heard the word, it didn't sink in what it might actually mean. The last time Chris had a biopsy was in September – when he was diagnosed with cancer. It should have triggered that memory for me, but what I heard and focused on was that everything was good.

With five days left until our wedding, we were bubbling with excitement, figuring out what we still needed to do when the phone rang. After Chris answered it, I watched him sit down slowly on his bed. His shoulders slumped and he propped his elbow on his knee and rested his head in his hand while he listened to whoever was talking to him. I couldn't see his face. He kept shaking his head and replied with one word answers, "Uh-huh" and "Okay." My hands turned into balls of fists and my heart started beating rapidly. I willed myself to stay calm.

"Okay, Steph and I will see you then," he said and hung up the phone.

See who? When? Where? What?

Chris fell back onto his pillow and rubbed his face. *Oh God, give us strength.* I sat next to him.

"What's wrong, Chris?" I whispered. He squeezed my hand while he continued to rub his forehead with the other. He sighed deeply, looking up at the ceiling, avoiding my eyes.

He looked devastated. No. He looked defeated.

"That was Dr. Chehval. The biopsy showed that there's another tumor."

What? It felt like I got slapped in the face. *Another tumor?*

"I can't believe it!" he yelled and punched the side of the bed. I grabbed him and held him in my arms for a long time. I felt a stream of warm, wet tears fall on my back and I prayed for strength and wisdom to help Chris. I don't know how I got the courage, but I knew God heard my prayer. I pulled back and cradled his face in my hands.

"Chris, we are going to keep fighting and we will beat this." He started to look down, but I held his face up. "I love you and I know you love me just as much. No matter what happens, nothing will ever take away our love. I'm not giving up, Chris, and neither are you. We are going to stay strong in our hope. God will help us find a way to beat this thing. Do you think that after all this time, when we finally found each other, that God would separate us? No. We will grow stronger in our love, in our faith in Him, and in our hope for your healing. We will have a family that we've always dreamed of and grow old together."

He looked at me and then kissed me deeply.

"I don't know what I've done to have someone like you in my life, but I am so blessed. I love you too, Steph, so very much. I'll do all I can to make you just as happy as you make me. Thank you for staying by my side. I'm not going to give up, ever."

God showed Chris and me that He is there with us in every moment – good and bad. We knew how much He loved us in the ways He helped us to be there for each other and how He worked through others to support us. Love always prevails. For it says,

"God sent His only Son into this world [so] *that we might have life through Him. This is love: not that we loved God but that He first loved us. No one has ever seen God, but if we love one another, God lives in us and His love spreads freely among us."*

- 1st John 4:9 – 10; 12.

His Word repeats this message as a reminder to us how much He loves us. Find more of these scriptures and let them build up your faith in your race.

"Live in faith and love, with endurance and gentleness. Fight the good fight of faith and win everlasting life to which you were called when you made the good profession of faith in the presence of so many witnesses."

- 1st Timothy 6:11 – 12

God is the Word. The Word is God. Spend time in the Word. Spend time with God. Turn to Him and pray. Focus on what God *can* do. You don't have to understand and it may not even make sense to you, but choose to trust Him. Be strong. Have faith. Hold on to your hope. Find the will and patience to wait on God.

"For humans it is impossible, but for God all things are possible."

- Matthew 19: 26

Like an athlete who trains for an upcoming race and practices his or her skill repeatedly, you, too, must also train in God's Word and meditate over it. The difference between you and the athlete is that you are not preparing for your race, you're already in it. The starting gun has been fired. So walk, run, or ride on with God on your side.

"If God is with us, then who shall be against us?"

- Romans 8:31

I found out we were meeting Dr. Chehval in the afternoon, a couple of hours before our wedding rehearsal. We didn't want to worry our families and closest friends so we agreed to tell them after our honeymoon. We promised each other that nothing would steal the joy from the happiest day of our lives.

When I arrived at the medical office building, Chris was already there, leaning against the wall, waiting for me. It brought me back to when we first met at the movie theater. I couldn't stop smiling and told him what I was thinking about.

"That's one of my top ten best moments," Chris said.

"Oh, and what is your number one?"

"It will be when you walk down that aisle," he whispered in my ear. I gazed into his soft, loving eyes and felt so much love in them, it made me shiver.

"Then it's date. Be at the church on Saturday, 2 p.m. sharp. I'll be the one in a white dress."

"Funny girl," he laughed.

While Dr. Chehval examined Chris, I tried to imagine what it would be like to see my groom for the first time. I hoped I would walk to the man of my dreams down that long aisle without tripping in my dress and be able to keep my composure through my vows to him.

"Stephanie," the receptionist called out, interrupting my thoughts, "you can go in now." I walked in Dr. Chehval's office and sat down next to Chris.

"The tumor is not in the urethra. It developed on the left side of the penis," Dr. Chehval began. "It's about the size of a small pea. We know the PET scan didn't show any cancerous activity above from where the tumor had been removed, but there were questions below the pelvic area. It's possible that the tumor was beginning to form and it couldn't be detected because of the scar tissue and inflammation within the area.

I suggest trying a cryosurgical technique. It's a process to freeze and defrost the tumor repeatedly using liquid nitrogen that would damage the cells inside the nodule. Then the body disposes of it."

"Okay, let's do it," Chris said. We found out that the surgery was scheduled a week after we would get back from our honeymoon.

"It's all going to be good, Steph."

"I know, Chris. I'm not worried."

"To hope is the way we are saved. But if we saw what we hoped for, there would no longer be hope: how can you hope for what is already seen? So, we hope for what we do not see and we will receive it through patient hope."

- Romans 8:24-25

Bliss

"If we love one another, God lives in us and His love is made perfect for us".

- 1st John 4:12

I woke up early the morning of our wedding day, but rather than get up, I took the time to think over everything, relishing the anticipation and excitement. I promised myself I would do all I could to cherish each moment and not let it go by so fast that I wouldn't remember it. I knew I could do this because I've done it before – without realizing it – so many years ago.

When I was around three-years-old, I couldn't hear anything unless it was very loud such as an airplane flying overhead or my dog barking in the house. My parents would find me plopped on the floor, in front of the television, pressing my ear against the speaker so I could hear it.

After a series of tests, the doctor discovered I was severely deaf. The day I put on my first hearing aid was a day I would never forget. I was sitting on my father's lap when I heard his deep, gruff voice for the first time.

"Can you hear me, baby girl?" he asked.

With wide eyes, I squeezed his cheeks and he repeated his question. I touched my ear and I laughed. My father smiled as tears inched slowly down his face. I felt a tug on my shirt and looked at my mother, asking if I could hear her too. I laughed again, hearing my parents for the first time. On the way home, I discovered a world of sounds, pointing to everything and wanting to know about it. I heard an ambulance siren wind its way through the streets. I felt the vibrations of an 18-wheeler and heard its giant wheels speeding by us on the highway.

When we got home, I jumped out of the car and ran into my house. I looked at my dog, jumping at my knees and heard her happy greeting. I fell to the floor laughing while she smothered my face with her excited kisses. I got up to look for my brother, Rich, and found him playing with his friends in the backyard and heard his laughter. I noticed the birds in our oak tree and discovered the sweet songs they made. I jumped when I heard the telephone ring. I ran all over the place, discovering the many different sounds and asking what they were. It was the happiest day of my life and I could remember it as if it just happened the day before.

Treasuring this memory, I laid there in bed and asked God to help me cherish each special moment of my wedding day so that I could remember every happy detail.

I found out later that Chris had gotten up early too and went on a bike ride, his first one since September. He wanted to feel the freedom on his bike again and rode about 25 miles. We were able to have a little time to ourselves to enjoy the peacefulness and the true meaning of the day that we had both waited for, for such a long time.

When our families and friends arrived at the church, everything flowed smoothly. People were putting decorations up in the church. Some of the ladies were pinning the flowers on the men's tuxedos. Our photographer was already busy taking pictures. Everyone worked together to make sure Chris and I didn't see each other before the ceremony. I surveyed the church and saw so many happy faces that I couldn't stop smiling and wondered if they were just as excited as Chris and I were.

When I returned to the dressing room, Kelly, who was my matron-of-honor, helped drape the back of my dress over several chairs behind me so I could sit and relax. After I checked my veil and make-up, I watched my bridesmaids fuss over their deep metallic red dresses. I loved seeing the different styles they chose that fit perfectly with their personality and figure. Looking around, I caught Kelly's eye.

"Are you okay?" she asked slowly.

"Yes. Why?"

"I just had to make sure, because you are the calmest bride I have ever seen." We heard a knock on the door and Father John walked into the room.

"Well Stephanie, are you ready?" he asked. I nodded eagerly, smiling.

"Good," he clapped his hands together, "it's time."

"Yes," I yelled, jumping up and knocking over the chairs behind me, "I'm getting married!" Shocked, everyone laughed and untangled my train from the chairs and straightened my dress for me.

"Okay," Father John said, surprised. "Let's get everyone lined up in the hall and we'll begin."

When I walked into the hall, all eyes were on me. Mark, Patrick, and Michael gave me a gentle hug and said how happy they were for Chris and me.

"Chris is doing okay, Stephanie," Mark whispered. "He can't wait to see you."

The music started and each couple walked into the church one at a time while I stood in the back between my mother and Grandpa Schoonover. I started to think about my father, wishing he was the one who could walk me down the aisle. I closed my eyes and imagined he was next to me. *Dad, I know you're here. I think you would approve of Chris and be proud of the kind of man he is and how good he is to me. I love you.* There was a sense of surreal peace and love in my heart and I knew I was feeling my father's presence. My mother tugged my arm, alerting me that it was time and I let her and Grandpa Schoonover escort me inside the church.

When we approached the long aisle, I was anxious to see Chris, but I suddenly felt a pull on my dress. First on my left and then on my right. I glanced down and realized my mother and grandfather were stepping on it. As we walked together, I was being pulled down on the left, then on the right and then at the same time. I bent my knees to lower myself and felt the strain of the dress pulling from my neck. I was afraid the buttons would snap open so I hung back to let them lead me and I was relieved from the heavy feet under me. I took several deep breaths to regroup and the moment I saw Chris, nothing else mattered. He stood tall and proud in his black tuxedo with his hands tightly folded in front of him. I couldn't take my eyes off him.

After my mother and grandfather handed me over to Chris, he wrapped my arm around his and squeezed my hand.

"Thank you for marrying me," he whispered in my ear.

"Thank you for asking me, Chris."

Father John talked to us about the significance and the commitment of marriage between a man and a woman. I tried to listen, but I was mesmerized by Chris' adoring eyes that were looking deeply into mine.

As I gaze upon you, I realized this was no accident – us finding each other. Someone had a hand in it. So here we stand before our Lord, with our hands joined as one, declaring our love for many years to come.

Stephanie M. Saulet

When it was time to share our vows, Chris repeated each line with confidence, assurance, and love and it gave me goose bumps all over my arms and legs. I felt so much love for Chris and from him that I struggled to enunciate each word of my vows to him. Chris stroked my fingers and squeezed my hands, encouraging me. I found his strength within me and continued.

"...in sickness and in health," I choked, catching my breath, "to love and to cherish until death us do part." I swallowed the lump in my throat. "I love you, Chris," I whispered, fighting back the tears.

"I love you, too," he said and winked.

We spent the next two days with Chris' family and preparing for our honeymoon to Jamaica. We wanted to go somewhere warm and tropical where life would slow down. For the first time in months, it was just the two of us. No doctors, no tests, no appointments, and no meetings. Every day, we lounged on the beach feeling the soft, gentle breeze swaying the branches in the palm trees and listening to the soft brushes of the waves against the shoreline. Sometimes we'd watch people swimming, parasailing, kayaking, and boogie boarding and other times we'd fall into the trance of the ocean and take naps.

One day, Chris surprised me with a couples' massage. We walked a small distance down the beach and found a hut all by itself perched on wooden posts. There were no windows, but the walls were high and you could only see the top of a person's head if he or she was tall like Chris. The roof was made of straw and dried palm tree branches. The set-up was as tropical as the scenery. The music was the ocean and an occasional call from a seagull. The scents were perfumed by the tropical flowers, mixed in with the sea salt. Chris and I became hypnotized by the setting as we gazed into each other's eyes during our massage. I felt like I was floating along the waves in Chris' strong arms holding me close to him. It was so serene and magical. I found out that Chris felt the same way and was amazed at the closeness we shared.

We enjoyed many ethnic delicacies from the resort since they hosted a different nationality each day, serving its specialties. It felt like we traveled around the world within a week, exploring a variety of tastes and smells. Chris discovered a barbeque hut and we picnicked on the beach, eating Jamaican Jerk chicken for lunch. After a couple of lazy days, we started working out again and participated in some of the activities at the resort. Chris talked me into doing a sexy legs contest

94

and the only way I'd do it was if he would join me. He was the only man in the contest, but it didn't bother him. He played up his part, strutting back and forth in front of the judges showing off his legs and even pulling up his swim shorts just above his tan line. He pointed his toes and did a squat to show off his toned muscles, teasing the ladies. They admired his legs so much that he won most of the votes in the contest. After collecting his prize, he suddenly swept me in his arms, dipped me and embraced me in a long kiss, making everyone around us whoop and holler.

"Yeah, baby, yeah," he laughed.

One day, the theme was Greece and the resort held Beach Olympics that involved a relay race on the beach, tug-of-war, the biggest splash in the pool, and a relay race in the pool that ended with a volleyball game. Competitive by nature, Chris just had to enter in the events. I took pictures and encouraged him on the sidelines. He won the relay race, beating guys half his age by several feet. He encouraged his team to pull hard and strong in the tug-of-war and they won. He wasn't able to make the biggest splash, but he definitely gave it his best effort running hard, jumping high in the air, and pulling his knees close to his body before landing in the water.

By mid-afternoon, all the points were tallied and Chris won overall for the men. As a winner, he had to model the different ways to wear a toga for a Greek Toga party later that evening. The presenter goaded him into taking off his T-shirt, which had many ladies screaming over his toned body. Chris kept shaking his head, laughing, while he strutted back and forth on the stage. Finally, he stood like a Greek god in the long white sheet, wearing sunglasses and stretched out his left arm above his head and made a fist with his right hand on his chest. He received a standing ovation.

Later in the week, we booked an excursion to Dunn's River Falls. When we got there, Chris suddenly grabbed my hand and pulled me into the icy cold water with him.

"YEAH!" he yelled out with his thumb up while I gritted my teeth, trying to smile for the camera's shot of us.

We hiked up the waterfall, forming a long human chain holding each other's hand for support on the slippery rocks. It was awesome to climb next to massive, forceful water falling over the rocks into the sea. It was the clearest and purest water I've ever been in. Once we were able to slide down a little slope that landed us into a small pool about three feet deep. After we finally climbed out of the last set of rocks, we turned around and saw just how steep the waterfall was and were amazed how we had climbed to the top from the bottom, together, holding hands with strangers, supporting each other.

Even though we had wonderful experiences, the best part of our honeymoon was being together all the time. We felt like we could be ourselves and be normal – no mention of cancer. Of the many moments we cherished, it was being in each other's arms when we fell asleep and when we woke up each morning that we loved the most, realizing again, one of our most precious dreams had finally came true.

I promise to love you every day. Let me always walk beside you in the sunlight or in the rain. Let me share your joys and care for you in times of pain. Let me be your best friend, lover, and confidant, for you are all I'll ever want.

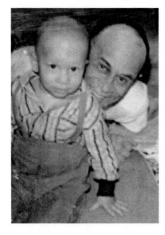

Chris with "Jamps." Chris loved his Grandfather very much.

With my favorite dolls.

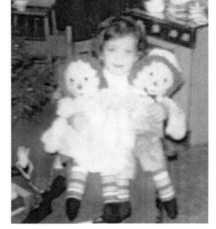

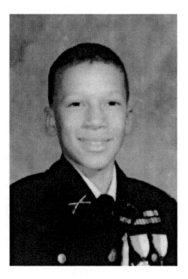

Chris in military school. It was the happiest time in his childhood.

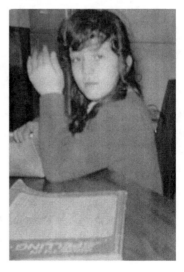

I was always studying. Spelling was my favorite subject.

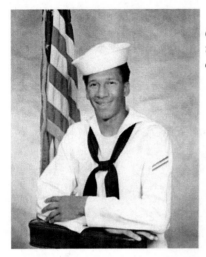

Chris in the U.S. Navy. He was proud to serve his country.

I loved dancing. I took lessons from when I was 3 to 15 years old.

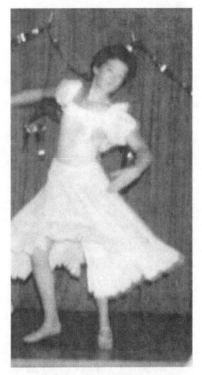

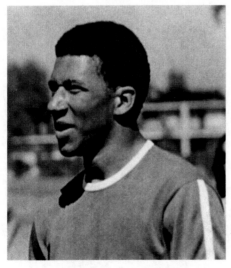

One of my favorite pictures of Chris.

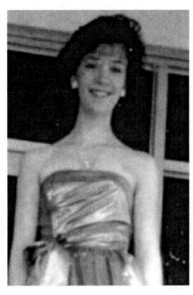

My High School Prom - 1990

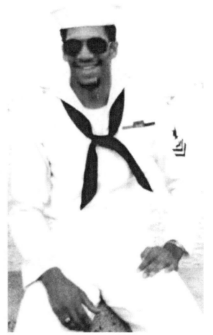

Chris loved traveling around the world in the Navy.

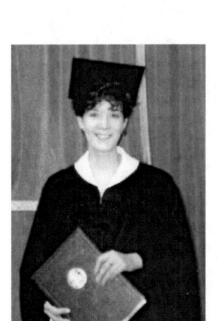

University of Missouri-St. Louis Graduate in 1995. I couldn't wait to start my teaching career.

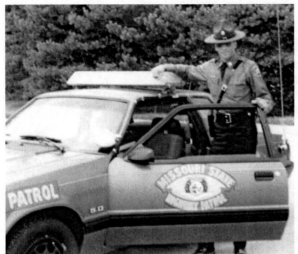

A proud trooper of the Missouri State Highway Patrol. Chris was promoted Sergeant in 1995.

Chris qualified for the St. Louis Team in Paris-Brest-Paris in 1999. He cycled 850 miles round trip in 86 hours. He was 40-years-old.

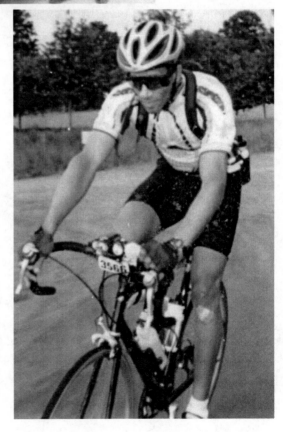

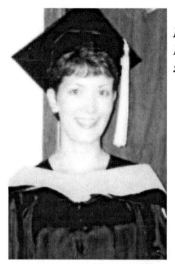

Master's Graduate from Lindenwood University, 2000.

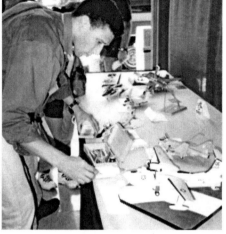

Chris' other passion was building military models since he was a young boy.

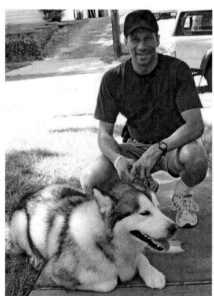

After the terrorist attack in 2001, Chris joined the Missouri Air National Guard.

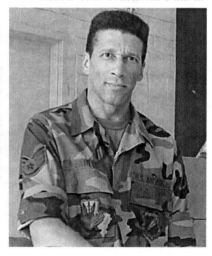

Chris and his dog, D'Artagnon.

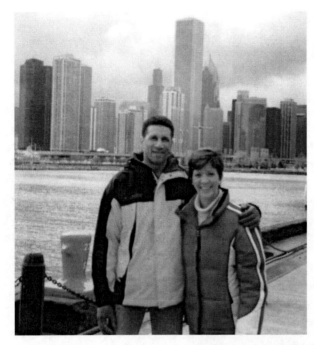

While we were
dating, we did a
lot of things
around town
and traveled
together.

Chicago - 2005

*I was selected as 1 of 10
teachers in St. Louis by
Boeing to attend Space
Camp for Teachers in
Huntsville, Alabama in
the summer of 2005. In
the picture, I was
Mission Specialist 2 on
my way to space to fix
the Hubble Telescope.
It was as close as I can
get to being an
astronaut!*

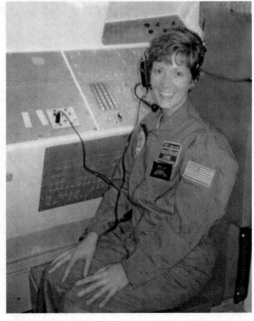

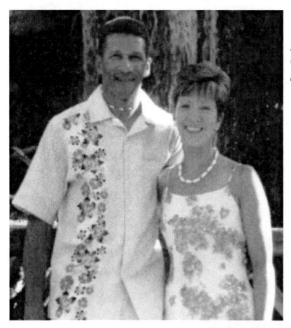

Engaged!
Oahu, Hawaii
Summer of 2005

Chris' last bicycle race
wearing a Momentum
jersey in September, 2005,
two weeks before the
cancer diagnosis.

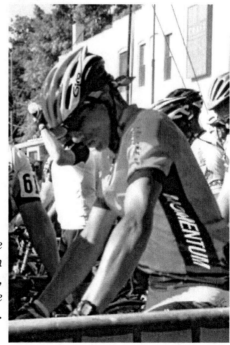

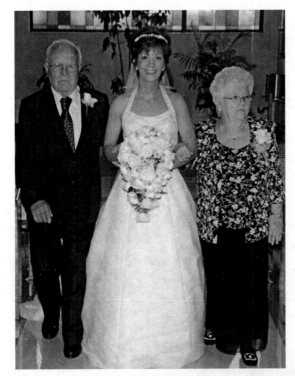

Grandpa Schoonover and my mother escorting me down the aisle to my groom.

(Courtesy of Photography by Daleen)

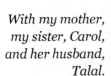

With my mother, my sister, Carol, and her husband, Talal.

(Courtesy of Photography by Daleen)

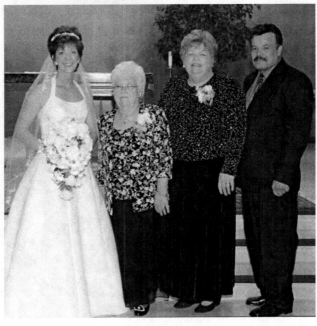

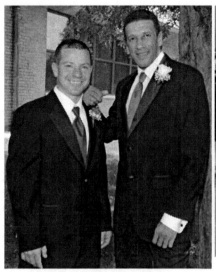

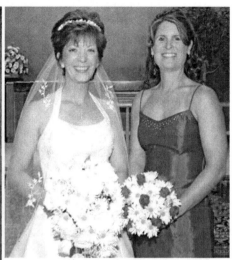

Hanging out with his best friend, Bob. (Courtesy of Photography by Daleen)

Best Girlfriends: with Kelly. (Courtesy of Photography by Daleen)

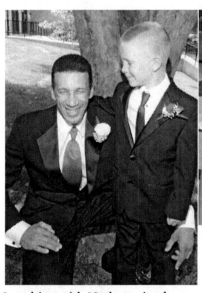

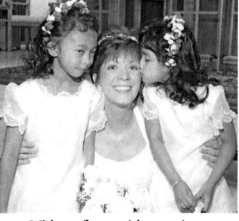

Laughing with Nathan, ring bearer. (Courtesy of Photography by Daleen)

With my flower girls, my nieces Celeste (left) and Nicole (right). (Courtesy of Photography by Daleen)

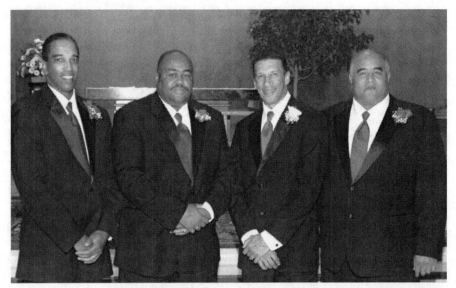

Proud Brothers (from left to right): Michael, Patrick, Chris, and Mark.
(Courtesy of Photography by Daleen)

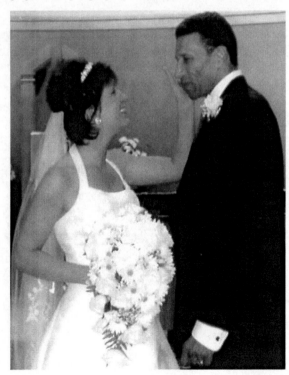

Sharing a moment.

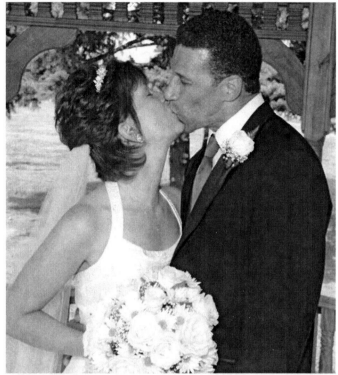

*Our special
kiss in the
gazebo.*

*(Courtesy of
Photography*

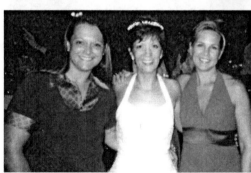

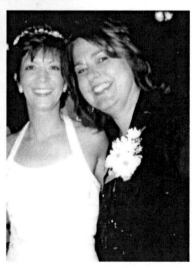

Top: with my 5ᵗʰ Grade Team, Ali (left)
and Amee (right)

Right: with Teddie Momma

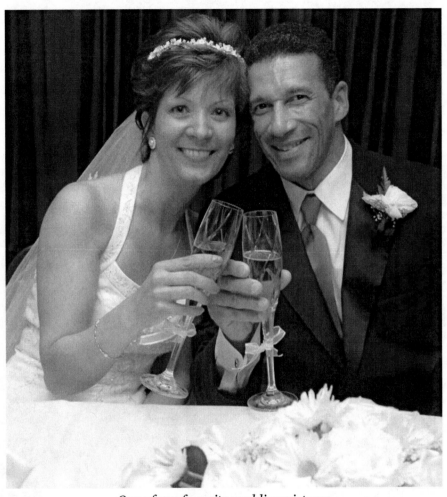

One of our favorite wedding pictures.

(Courtesy of Photography by Daleen)

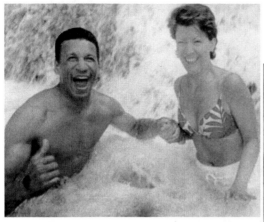

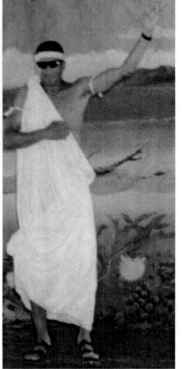

On our honeymoon in Jamaica.

Top: We just jumped in the icy cold water at Dunn's River Falls.

Right: Chris posing as a Greek god.

Bottom: Romantic dinner on the resort.

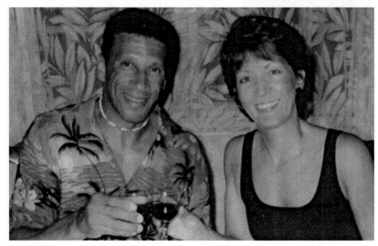

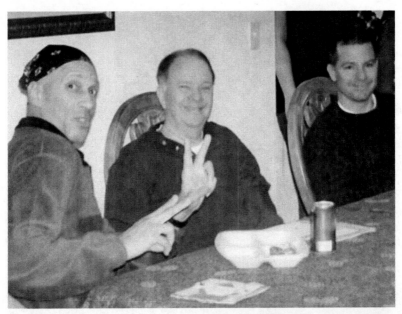

*Top: Chris with Poppa
Bob and Bob.
Christmas – 2006*

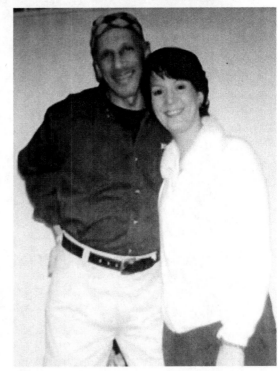

*Right: Our first
Christmas as husband
and wife - 2006*

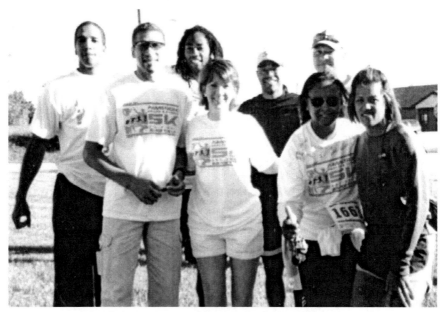

Tour de Troy – 2007 (from left) with Michael,
Mark Jr., Darren, Rich, Toni, and Verisha.

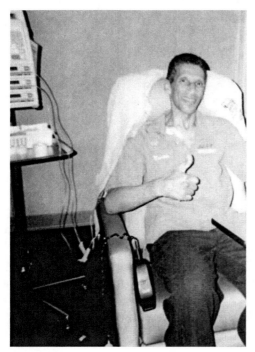

"This one is going to work,
Steph!" Chris said each
time we tried a new chemo
regimen.

Spring – 2008

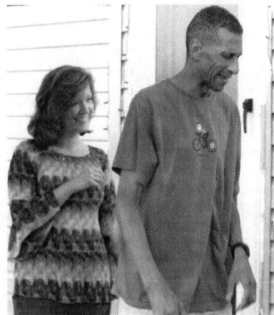

Left: Chris' 50th Birthday Party, October - 2008

I think I succeeded in surprising him!

Below: Our last picture together. Christmas – 2008, two weeks before hospice care.

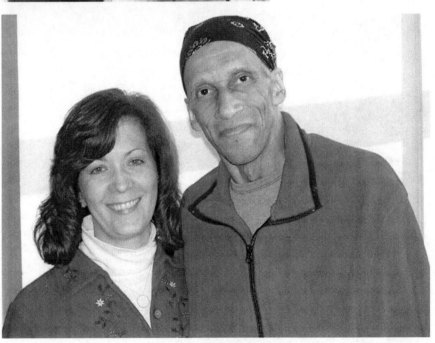

Back in the Race

Corners are like blind spots on the road, you can't see around them. But to keep on going, it takes faith and courage to turn into the corners anyway.

After we came home, Chris didn't waste any time getting back into his fight and we saw Dr. Chehval for a follow-up. During the exam, he discovered another lump that was most likely another tumor Chris hadn't noticed before. It was smaller than its counterpart. Dr. Chehval told us that he would do the cryosurgical procedure on both tumors. If everything goes well, he would attempt to reconstruct the urethra and Chris' face lit up.

"Sounds good to me, Doctor," he said optimistically.

We had a lot to do within the week of the surgery. We unpacked our suitcases and our wedding gifts. I organized our house and worked on the thank you notes while Chris returned to work for a few days. We were finding our new norm and adjusting easily to our married life and we couldn't be happier.

We talked about the procedure and prayed that it would work against the tumors. We felt our energy had been re-charged while we were away and felt stronger coming into this next leg of the race.

"Let us hold fast to our hope without wavering, because He who promised is faithful."

- Hebrews 10:23

We checked in at the surgery center early in the morning and began preparing Chris for the procedure. He was in good spirits and anxious to get started, checking his watch every several minutes. Fortunately, the day's schedule was on time but it wasn't soon enough for Chris whose stomach emitted a low rumbling growl. He glanced at me with the pained look of a hungry little boy and I had to laugh.

"I'm sorry Chris, but your facial expressions can be too cute sometimes."

Dr. Chehval came by to review Chris' chart. He told some of his team who were with him that he and his wife came to our wedding and complimented us on our beautiful ceremony.

"It really meant a lot to us that you came, Doctor," Chris said, stretching his hand out to him. "Thank you."

After signing Chris' chart, Dr. Chehval told him that he'd see him soon and he would talk to me afterwards. Dr. Faller sat down next to Chris and re-assessed his IV.

"Well, Chris, it's about that time, so give your bride a kiss before I inject the happy medicine in your IV."

"What? I'm already happy," he said, smiling.

"Me too," I whispered and kissed my husband goodbye.

"Stephanie, we'll take good care of him," Dr. Faller promised, "and Dr. Chehval will send word to you when we have begun the procedure."

Watching them take Chris away from me, I felt a heavy weight bear down in my chest. I wished I could be near him, just to hold his hand. I prayed to God to watch over Chris and to guide Dr. Chehval's hands skillfully and successfully during the surgery.

In the waiting room, I focused on God's magnificent, graceful hands guiding Dr. Chehval's while he operated on Chris. I imagined the peacefulness in Chris' body, mind, and spirit knowing God was in control. I sat there alone, but I was not lonely.

"As for me, I watch in hope for the Lord, I wait for God, my Savior. My God will hear me."

- Micah 7:7

I felt God's presence deep within me and I knew He was also there in the operating room. I began to feel peaceful and a strong power of hope.

"May our Lord Jesus Christ, who has loved us, and may God our Father, who in His mercy gives us everlasting comfort and true hope, strengthen you."

- 2nd Thessalonians 2:16

I didn't realize Dr. Chehval was sitting next to me until I felt his hand on mine and I jumped when I opened my eyes. He smiled.

"Chris is already in the recovery room and is doing fine. The procedure went well and everything looked good. I began with the cryosurgical technique on the two nodules and it will be a matter of time before Chris' body will dispose of them. Then I checked his bladder and assessed the sphincter muscle and showed no signs of cancer."

Thank you, God!

"I was able to reconstruct the urethra and inserted a catheter through it. Chris will have to tolerate the catheter for about two weeks

114

or so to allow time for his body to adjust to the reconstruction and to prevent any scar tissue from developing inside the new urethra. He will be in the hospital for about two days. I know he gets easily stressed staying here, so the sooner I can release him to rest at home the better it will be for him and for you."

I hugged Dr. Chehval and thanked him for giving Chris a chance. He promised to stop by later to check on him. I called our families and close friends to tell them the good news God granted us. Once I got word about Chris' room number, I went and organized his things for him. Filled with anxious excitement, I couldn't wait to see him and paced back and forth until I saw Chris being pushed into the room. He was wide awake and alert.

"Hey pretty lady," he greeted. I gave him a quick kiss and was told to step out in the hall so the nurse could help him get settled in the bed and assess his vitals. When I walked back into the room, Chris was all smiles.

"Did you see Dr. Chehval?" he asked. Before I could answer, he continued. "Everything went well, Steph. The cancer is destroyed and I'm healed. Thank God," he shouted, pumping his fists high in the air. "It's all good, Steph," he said, patting the side of the bed for me to sit next to him. "I love you so much."

"The Lord is my strength and my shield; my heart trusts in Him, and I am helped. My heart leaps for joy and I will give thanks to Him!"
- Psalm 28:7

After two days in the hospital, Chris was released. It felt so good to bring him home and it was even better that I could stay with him and not have to leave anymore.

After several days of recuperating, Chris felt strong enough to enjoy the Fourth of July with our neighbors. I couldn't tell who was happier, Chris or his friends, being able to hang out together again. They knew he was still a little beat from the surgery and did all they could to make him feel comfortable, especially in the warm July heat. They carried our two-seater swing over from our house and put it in the shade for Chris.

One of the neighbors remembered when Chris brought me over two years before at their Fourth of July gathering and introduced me to them for the first time. She leaned over and whispered in my ear,

"I knew you were the one for Chris. I'm so happy for the both of you."

We talked about our wedding reception, remembering how Chris and I danced the night away and how much fun we had.

"Do you realize that this is this first time we are with our neighbors as a married couple?" he asked, smiling. "I'm loving every minute of it being here with my wife." Watching Chris enjoy his friends, being so happy, I realized this was the way it should be for us. I thanked God again for blessing us with so much joy and love between us, our families, and our friends.

Throughout the rest of the week, Chris endured the catheter as well as he could, although it caused him a lot of discomfort and irritation. But he never complained. One day over the weekend, he walked into the living room with a huge grin on his face.

"Steph," he paused and I glanced up at him, wondering what was up. "I can't feel the tumors anymore." It took a moment before I understood the significance of what he said and jumped up.

"Oh my God, Chris. God is so good!" I shouted with tears of joy streaming down my face. Chris laughed and held me tight against him.

"I can't wait to tell Dr. Chehval on Monday morning. We have a lot to look forward to, Steph."

"'I know the plans I have for you; plans to prosper you and not harm you; plans to give you hope and a future,' declares the Lord."
- Jeremiah 29:11

Challenges

When you turn into that corner and discover the detours up ahead, you can choose to quit or dig deep within yourself to ride on through them.

When we saw Dr. Chehval that Monday morning, he told us the tumors had dissolved and we were all exhilarated that the procedure worked. Dr. Chehval wanted to do a cystoscopy at the end of the week to see how the reconstructed urethra was healing before deciding to remove the catheter. Looking down, Chris pressed his lips together.

"Chris," Dr. Chehval said and he looked up at his doctor, "I know you're disappointed, thinking I'd remove the catheter today. I want to be sure first. Try to be patient and give your body the time it needs to fully heal."

When we walked out of the office, Chris was still quiet.

"No worries, babe," I said. He smiled slightly. "It's all going to work out," I reminded him. After a few more steps, he nodded.

Oh God, give us the strength we both need to get through the rest of this week. Help ease Chris' discomfort from the catheter.

By Saturday morning, Chris was more than ready to have the catheter removed. He was irritable and cranky, abruptly responding to the same questions with short answers and asking how long it would take before the procedure. This was not like him and some staff members who worked with him several times were surprised by his temperament, but they empathized with him by being patient and offering words of encouragement. After going through the pre-op routine so many times already, I wondered if either of us would ever get used to it. How could anyone get used to putting their life in someone else's hands? I realized it was a constant reminder to us that we do not always have control over our lives. We needed to keep our focus on the One who is always in control.

"If God is with us, who can be against us?"

- Romans 8:31

I kissed my husband goodbye and stood in the middle of the empty hallway, watching him disappear into the operating room – a scene I was intimately familiar with – and each time loneliness would attack my heart. I asked God to take it from me and let me feel His loving comfort. I walked into the vacant waiting room and once again, I wasn't alone. I felt a sense of calmness and thanked God for hearing my prayer. I didn't have to wait long when Dr. Chehval met up with me.

"Everything looked good. There was some scar tissue that I cleaned up, but the reconstructed urethra is healing nicely." He paused. "Stephanie, I'm not comfortable removing the catheter yet. I feel Chris needs more time for his body to heal."

"I understand, but it's been 17 days and he's so miserable with it."

"I know it's very uncomfortable for him, but I want to give his body enough time to heal in order to prevent any scar tissue from growing inside the urethra. Otherwise it would defeat the purpose of the reconstruction and cause more problems for Chris. This is only temporary," he said, tapping my hand.

"You're right, but try and tell Chris." Dr. Chehval promised to talk to him when the anesthesia wore off. I gave God thanks that Chris was healing well and asked for the patience we both needed to accept the time it would take for his body to fully heal.

When I heard my name, I slowly walked to Chris' room, nervous about what kind of attitude I would encounter from him. I opened his door carefully and peeked in. He was staring at the ceiling with a somber expression on his face.

"Chris?"

"Dr. Chehval didn't remove the catheter," he said somberly.

I've never experienced a catheter and I had no idea how unbearable it could be to tolerate. So, I couldn't tell him I understood or I knew what he was going through to comfort him. *God, what should I say to help him?*

"Chris," I whispered again, "but we have good news – you *are* healing. Isn't that what we prayed for? Let's focus on that to get through this."

He was quiet for awhile, still avoiding my eyes. I knew he was thinking it over and I had to wait until he was ready to talk about it.

"Okay, Steph," he said, finally meeting my eyes.

"Okay, what?"

"I'm not going to let this get the best of me," he smiled.

"He makes firm the steps of those who delight in Him. They may stumble, but they will not fall, for the Lord holds them by the hand."
                                                                          - Psalm 37:23 – 24

Three days later, we met with Dr. Chehval for a follow-up appointment. He still didn't remove the catheter and wanted to wait another week. I squeezed Chris' hand firmly.

"Remember, we're not going to let this get the best of us," I reminded him.

"Okay, we'll see you next week," he said and shook Dr. Chehval's hand.

While I was making the appointment for us, Chris rummaged around the candy bowl for a root beer sucker. He found it and a grape one too.

"You are such a kid, Chris." I laughed.

"Hey, I always get a sucker whenever I leave the doctor's office. I've been doing this since I was little boy."

"But you're only supposed to take one."

"Aw, come on. I was especially good today. Don't I deserve two suckers?"

"I'd say he does," Dr. Chehval said, overhearing our conversation. Chris popped a sucker in his mouth with a goofy grin and winked.

Over the next week, Chris took each day one at a time, tolerating the catheter and enduring the painful discomfort from it. He stayed busy working on one of his model projects and I had to begin setting up my classroom for a new school year. It was hard to believe that summer was almost over and I was beginning to wonder how I could be there for my husband and for my students.

When we returned to Dr. Chehval, he decided to remove the catheter with the condition Chris would return in two days for a re-evaluation. After 27 days with it, Chris was finally free. One more thing that would have made this day perfect for him would have been to ride his bicycle again.

One of Chris' proudest accomplishments was qualifying to ride for the St. Louis Team in the Paris-Brest-Paris race in 1999. Training for this competition required him to ride hundreds of miles to build up his strength and endurance. Early on Sunday mornings, he would get up when he knew there would be minimal traffic and ride his bike from St. Charles to downtown St. Louis, grab lunch, and then ride back. It was this incredible discipline and commitment to achieving his goal that won him a place on the team.

In order to succeed in the race, the cyclist would have to ride 850 miles in 90 hours. At 40-years-old, Chris was able to complete it in 86 hours. He remembered his shoulders and neck being so tensed that he and a teammate tied a rope from his helmet to the back of his seat just to keep his head up. He became so fatigued that he fell asleep while riding and tumbled over on his bike, banging up his knee on the gravel. It never crossed his mind to quit. He dug deep within himself to find the mental and physical strength to ride on. He visualized and focused on the finish line and knew he would cross over it on his bike victoriously within the time-frame of the race.

I believe this experience became his hallmark in the race for his life – fighting the cancer for as long as he did. He kept his focus on the finish line determined to cross over it victoriously.

Feeling the freedom from the catheter, Chris couldn't stop smiling as he bounced out of Dr. Chehval's office.

"Soon, Steph, I'll be back on the bike and riding again," he said confidently. "But in the meantime, guess what I'm going to do as soon as we get home?" I looked at him questionably. "I'm going to play with D'Artagnon and take him on a short walk." I wanted to tell him he should take it easy and let his body recuperate, but I couldn't.

About 36 hours later, Chris started having some problems voiding. I wondered if it was the scar tissue Dr. Chehval worried about. I felt that our patience was being tried, and prayed for perseverance to be patient during Chris' recovery.

"By faith, we have received true righteousness and we are at peace with God. We feel secure, even in our trials, knowing that trials produce patience, from patience comes merit, merit is the source of hope, and hope does not disappoint us because the Holy Spirit has been given to us, pouring into our hearts the love of God."

- Romans 5:1, 3 – 5

The next morning, we were back at Dr. Chehval's office, still feeling hopeful. After examining Chris, we found out that there was some scar tissue developing inside the reconstructed urethra and Chris would have to tolerate the catheter again. Dr. Chehval wanted us to return first thing the next morning at the surgery center to re-insert the catheter. Chris was very quiet after we left the office and I knew enough to let him be so that he could deal with it in his own way.

After a couple of days adjusting to the catheter again, Chris had a new sense of energy. He kept busy with his models, played with his dog, helped me with the chores and errands, and started walking on the treadmill again. There were no more excuses, in Chris' opinion, to slow down or not do the things he knew he could do himself even though he had to do it with the catheter. He decided to go to the IPMS convention in Kansas City for several days. He needed to get away and wanted to enjoy his hobby that he loved so much. I was amazed how he managed with the catheter while he scouted the vending tables, sold some of his kits and supplies, studied and judged the models and dioramas entered in the contest, and traded tips and skills with others. No one knew that he had just fought a battle with cancer or that he was tolerating a catheter. He seldom talked about himself except to proudly introduce me as his wife to his friends. By the weekend, I noticed Chris was getting worn out and was beginning to feel uncomfortable again. When it was time to load up his kits, models, and supplies, he couldn't do it and accepted help from others. I admired his humility and grace as he thanked everyone for their help.

On the way home, I began to feel the nervousness and anticipation of going back to work for the new school year. *How am I going to be able to divide my time teaching and doing my job and be there for Chris in the way he needed me?* I felt like I was in the middle of a tug-of-war between the two. There is so much to do as a full-time teacher such as following each subject's curriculum and lesson plans, training and workshops, collaboration with colleagues and my principal, staff and district meetings, communication with parents, and constant evaluation of students' progress. All of these take up a lot of time outside the classroom, and Chris still needed me by his side more than before. *How am I going to do it all?*

A sense of panic mixed with fear began to cloud my mind and I had no clue how to work it out. I did the only thing I knew to do, I prayed. I asked God for the strength He knew I would need to get through this next leg of the race. For it says,

"My flesh and my heart may fail; but God is the strength of my heart."

- Psalm 73:26

I woke up that Monday morning, feeling sick to my stomach, I couldn't eat my breakfast. I wanted to go with Chris to his appointment with Dr. Chehval, but it was my first contractual day of the school year.

"Hey, no worries, Steph," he said, holding me. "I'm going to be okay. Everything will work out." Even though I didn't tell Chris about my thoughts returning to work, he could read me so well. I held him tightly, not wanting to let him go. I told him that I would call him during my first break.

I took many deep breaths driving to school and kept praying for that strength I needed. I realized if I could get through the first day, then maybe the next day would be a little easier. Fortunately, I was so busy and distracted in the meetings that the morning flew by. When I had a break, I grabbed my cell phone and called Chris, anxious to know what happened at his appointment. When I heard his voice, I could tell things didn't go well. He still had to tolerate the catheter for another week.

"Hang in there, Chris. Just keep remembering that you're not going to let this get the better of you," I encouraged.

When I came home, Chris looked worn out sitting on the couch. Sometime after we talked, he had some problems with the catheter. He started feeling pressure in his bladder and had to return to Dr. Chehval, who relieved the pressure for Chris. However, he needed a new catheter and would have to have another out-patient procedure to replace it.

God, how much more could this man take?

I tried to reassure Chris to get through this one day at a time and try to be patient for his body to heal.

Out of the blue, Chris exploded, "I have been patient! But how much longer do I have to wear a catheter? Everyday, I'm patient and dealing with this thing without complaining. I'm doing everything I'm supposed to do to get better. I was supposed to be back at work and getting back on my bike by now. I don't know how to fix this, and I don't know how much more of this I can take. It's so uncomfortable and painful – especially when I move, sit down, lie down or stand up again. I can't even relax enough to do anything! I have to re-adjust this tube with the bag and my pants every time I move. It's humiliating and I'm tired of this, Steph."

I felt my husband's exasperated frustration and I had no idea what I could say to make it better. *Please, give Chris relief. Give us the strength we both need to get through this. God, please take his pain away.*

"I'm sorry I blew up. I guess I just needed to vent and you're here with me. I actually feel better now. Thanks for listening."

We talked about how we could help each other be patient while his body healed and prayed for the strength we needed to get through each day.

A couple of days later, Chris went through the procedure with no problems. Dr. Chehval found more scar tissue in the urethra and cleared it out. He didn't want to take a chance of any more scar tissue blocking it as Chris' body continued to heal. We focused on the good news even though Chris still had to put up with the catheter longer.

"The Lord is my strength, my shield; in Him, my heart trusts."

- Psalm 28:7

Pothole from Hell

When you get to the point when you think you can't take the pain from the race anymore, it becomes a moment when you discover your true inner strength.

The follow-up appointment after the procedure went well even though Chris still had to put up with the catheter. Little by little, things were starting to get better. Chris continued doing things around the house and worked on his model projects without any problems. I was getting to know my students and establishing a successful routine with them during our first week of school. We made the best of our time together in the evenings, talking about our day and just being with each other.

We grew more hopeful that things were turning around. It felt like we were riding with momentum along this flat stretch.

Suddenly, we hit a huge pothole out of nowhere. It was almost like Chris' bicycle accident several years before we met. In that accident, he was enjoying the thrill of gliding down a hill at about 35 to 40 mph and when he rounded the corner, his front tire hit a pothole. He flipped over with his bike and crashed on the pavement, ripped up in several places, but still alive.

That was how it felt at the end of the week.

After school was dismissed, I checked my cell phone for messages and found out Chris was being admitted into the surgery center, but I didn't know why. I called him back and only got his voice mail. I grabbed my things and raced out of the building. Despite my attempts to stay calm, I felt a surge of panic. My heart was pounding so hard, it was difficult to breathe. *Oh God, please let Chris be okay.*

I pulled into the garage across from the surgery center and kept circling around to find a parking spot. When I finally found one, I struggled to put my car in Park. It went into Reverse, then Drive, then Neutral. *Oh for crying out loud, park the damn thing.* My hands were shaking so hard, I couldn't put the car in the right gear. When I finally had it in Park, I yanked the keys out of the ignition, snatched my purse from the passenger seat, jumped out and slammed the door, creating a dull echo through the garage. I didn't look for any oncoming cars and took off running across the street like a rabbit escaping from D'Artagnon's jaws, through the doors, and up to the information desk. I asked in exasperated breaths where my husband, Christopher Saulet was. After several minutes of waiting (which felt like an hour) for the lady to give me the information I desperately needed, she told me that he was already in the surgical pre-op area. She started to tell me how to get there, when I swirled around and dashed through the closed doors. I ran down the hall and rounded the corner into the room.

"Can I help you?" a nurse asked. I ignored her and found Chris at the far end of the room, laying on a gurney with his fists clenched and eyes closed. I quickly went to him, dropped my things on a chair, took a deep breath and touched his hand.

"I'm here, Chris," I whispered, out of breath.

"Excuse me ma'am, but you are not supposed to..." I cut her off.

"I'm Christopher's wife and I am staying with my husband." She nodded and walked away.

"I'm glad you're here," Chris said, struggling to get his words out. He squeezed my hand hard and with his other hand, grabbed his head. *Oh God, help him.*

He let out a deep sigh and told me what was going on.

"The pressure started building up in my bladder again. Dr. Chehval is on vacation, so I went in to see Dr. Hoffman, but he wasn't able to relieve it, which is why I'm here."

"I'm so sorry you have to go through this," I whispered. He squeezed my hand again and closed his eyes tightly as he felt another round of spasms from his bladder. I wanted to get someone to help him, but his grip was so hard, I couldn't move.

A tall, thin bald man in a white doctor's coat appeared and checked Chris' file.

"You must be Chris' wife, Stephanie." I nodded. "I'm Dr. Hoffman."

I was in no mood to be cordial.

"Doctor, Chris is in so much pain, can you please do something for him?"

"We're ready for him now," he said, as an anesthesiologist – one we didn't know – came up to Chris and re-assessed his IV while Dr. Hoffman explained that he would remove the scar tissue, re-insert a new catheter, and then talk to me afterwards. He turned around and left while the anesthesiologist injected a dose of the medicine, but this time there were no jokes or laughter – only pain and stress.

"I love you, Chris. It'll all be over soon," I whispered and suddenly he was wheeled away from me. The nurse I was rude to earlier told me that I could wait for my husband in the post-op room where they would bring him after the recovery. I nodded, still staring down the hall. I didn't know what to do or, for the moment, even how to walk. I just stood there like I was frozen. The nurse turned me around and guided me to Chris' post-op room and pointed to the information desk if I needed anything. She wished me luck and left me there in the doorway.

Within the last half hour, everything fast-forwarded: my heart, my mind, my body, the urgency of getting to my husband, and the desperation to relieve his pain and then suddenly things were at a stand-still. There was no screeching of the tires to slow down. It was like hitting that pothole and when you crash, everything stops.

For the second time since Chris told me he had cancer, I was really scared. I knew I needed to calm down, so I sank in the chair in the dark room with only the florescent light from the hallway shining through the doorway. I took deep breaths – inhaling slowly through my nose and exhaling out of my mouth, reminding myself that God is the light that shines through the darkness.

[For Jesus said,] "I have come into the world as light, so that whoever believes in me may not remain in darkness."

- John 12:46

I began to pray for God to work through Dr. Hoffman so he could help my husband. I didn't know anything about him other than Chris had seen him a couple of times when Dr. Chehval was out. On those occasions, he was comfortable with him, so I put my trust in God that he would take good care of my husband in the same way that Dr. Chehval had always done.

Not knowing how much time had passed, I glanced at the clock on the wall and saw that a half-an-hour had gone by. It usually took Dr. Chehval about this long, but since it was Dr. Hoffman's first time doing this procedure on Chris, he might take his time.

Another 15 minutes passed and still no word.

I turned on the television for some distraction, but I couldn't focus. So I turned it off and paced around the room, stopping at the doorway to find someone who could tell me what was going on. But each time, the hallway was deserted. *Where is everybody?* I looked at the clock again and noticed it had been 75 minutes. I was done waiting.

Doing my best to control my rising hysteria, I hurried over to the information desk and asked the nurse if she had heard anything about Chris. She hadn't and tried to encourage me to be patient. Exasperated, I slapped my hands down on the desk.

"This type of procedure normally takes a-half-an-hour and it has been *over* an hour. I *have* been patient and I want to know what is going on with my husband. *Now!*"

She nodded and slowly walked down the hall and disappeared. I stood there and waited for what seemed like forever when she finally returned and told me that Chris was still in surgery and Dr. Hoffman would talk to me afterward.

"Still in surgery? I don't understand."

"I'm sorry," she said sympathetically, "but that's all I know at this time. Dr. Hoffman will talk to you as soon as it's over."

Frustrated and confused, I walked back to the empty room and sat in the chair again. I wrapped my arms around myself, trying desperately to hold it together.

I tried not to look at the time again, but I couldn't help it. It was the only source of information I had. It had been 90 minutes since the surgery began. *Just breathe, Stephanie, breathe. Remember what Chris always says, "No worries, trust God."*

Feeling nauseous, I hunched over, fighting the fear threatening inside me. But I couldn't ignore it anymore: something was wrong – terribly wrong. *Oh God, please be with Chris. Take care of him. Guide Dr. Hoffman to do what is best for him. Let Chris be okay.*

It had been almost two hours when I noticed a shadow in the doorway. I looked up and saw Dr. Hoffman in light blue scrubs. I started to stand up, but he asked me to sit down with him. I searched his face for a sign of what he might say. His expression gave nothing away, taking off his cap and rubbing his perspiring head. I felt a lump form in my throat and I couldn't speak.

"Chris is doing fine and is in the recovery room," he said.

I felt my breath as it left my lungs, but something was not right. I clasped my hands tightly between my legs as he cleared his throat.

"There were complications," he paused.

"Com... complications?" I whispered. He nodded. *Oh God, help me.*

"I couldn't dilate the urethra because of the amount of scar tissue within the area. I tried repeatedly to clear it, but it was very tough and difficult. I consulted with the surgical team and I had no other choice but to insert a suprapubic catheter so Chris could still relieve himself." He paused to give me a moment to process everything.

"I don't understand," I choked, afraid to hear what he would say next.

"I had to create an opening just below Chris' belly button into the bladder and insert the catheter through the opening there," he said showing me on his stomach.

Oh... my... God! I felt the effects of hitting that pothole, remembering what Dr. Croft had told us months ago when we saw him for a second opinion. I couldn't speak and the tears flowed freely down my face.

"Do you have any questions?" he asked. I looked at him unable to speak over the lump in my throat.

He told me that the nurses would teach us how to handle a suprapubic catheter and we would have a follow-up appointment with Dr. Chehval next week. I was so overwhelmed that I just nodded, not fully comprehending anything. He left quietly and I was alone again in the dark, with only the light from the hallway beaming into the room.

What is this suprapubic catheter? What does it look like? How will this affect Chris' mobility? How serious is the scar tissue problem that resulted to using this type of catheter? Oh God. How? What? Why?

Questions, questions, questions – and no answers. But I knew God had the answers. I bowed my head low and prayed deeply. *Lord, help me. Show me Your strength, because I'm not strong enough. Tell me what to say to my husband. I love him so much, God. I know you love him too. Let us both feel Your presence within us and all around us.* I sat in the chair and rocked myself for a long time, waiting for what was to come for us.

"I'm down, but I'm not out. Though I sit in darkness right now, but the Lord is my light, and He will bring me out into the light."

- Micah 7:8 – 9

When the nurses brought Chris into the room, I quickly wiped my eyes, stood up, and straightened my shoulders back so I would at least appear strong for Chris.

When they began to transfer Chris from the gurney onto the hospital bed, his body started shaking uncontrollably.

"What's happening? Why is he shaking like that?" I cried, but no one answered.

"Wait," Chris pleaded, "Wait, please wait. There's something wrong here," he pointed toward his belly button. I fought back the tears, realizing he didn't know what it was yet. When one of the nurses told him, his eyes widened with fear and he looked at me, confused.

"Chris, listen to me," I said firmly. "It's okay. Do you hear me? You are okay."

He closed his eyes and started to calm down as the nurses helped him get settled into the bed, but he couldn't stop shaking. The other nurse explained that it could be the effects of the anesthetics since he did have some food earlier in the day, or it could be his body was in shock. I looked at her, stunned and prayed again for that strength we both needed to get through this.

"I cry out loudly to God, loudly I plead for mercy. I cried to my God for help; and He heard my voice"

- Psalm 18:7

After the nurses left, I walked over to Chris and stroked his forehead. The shakiness finally subsided and he started calming down, but there was still fear in his eyes that tore at my heart.

"Steph," he choked, "what's happened to me? What is it that I'm feeling here?" he asked, pointing to the suprapubic catheter.

I took a deep breath and slowly explained what Dr. Hoffman told me. As hard as I tried, I couldn't make my voice sound strong and I couldn't stop the tears. He kept shaking his head and I tried to assure him that things would be alright. He pushed my hand away and rubbed his forehead, trying to process everything. Suddenly, I saw a look on my husband's face that I had never seen before. It made me shiver and I felt immediately cold. It was a look of defeat. *My God, please don't let Chris give up. I am not going to give up and I don't want him to. Show me what to do to help my husband. Give us the strength we need, God. We can't fight this without you.* I just stood there. I couldn't find my voice and even if I had, I didn't know what I could say to make it better for him. So I waited again. I waited for Chris. I waited for God.

After some time had passed, Chris took my hand and brought it to his lips.

"Okay," he sighed. "Let's deal with this."

"... as for me, I am not giving up. I'm sticking around to see what God will do. I'm waiting for God to make things right. I'm counting on God to listen to me"

- Micah 7:7

After writing this, I realized that God was there, helping us. I truly believe He held us in the palm of His hand, carrying us while He renewed our strength to continue on in our journey together. For it says,

"I have chosen you and have not cast you away, fear not, for I am with you; be not dismayed, for I am your God. I will give you strength, I will bring you help, and I will uphold you with my right hand."

- Isaiah 41:9, 10, 13

So, if you ever feel like you're at the end of your rope, hang on and take a moment to know God is there with you.

"Be still and know that I am God."

- Psalm 46:10

Over the next several days, Chris learned how to adjust to the suprapubic catheter in the way he walked, sat, laid down, took a shower, and how to change the bandages around the incision and the tube. He started wearing loose baggy pants with no belt – something he had to get used to – but he needed to feel comfortable while concealing the catheter. Through all of this, what was most amazing to me was the way he coped. Every day he'd say,

"This too shall pass," with a wink and a smile that could melt butter.

He didn't let it stop him from living his life. He continued to work on his models, did errands and household chores while I worked, and played with D'Artagnon. Chris made the best of what he had to deal with and kept riding on in his race.

After a week with the new catheter, I went with Chris to see Dr. Chehval. After examining Chris, he assured us that Dr. Hoffman had done all he could to remove the scar tissue and if he was the surgeon, he would have made the same decision to insert the suprapubic catheter. There was no other way around it to help Chris relieve himself under those circumstances. I guessed this was supposed to make us feel better, but I still felt those intense emotions that I had during that hour-and-a-half of waiting. I never told Chris about it and I knew it was something I had to work through myself.

Over Labor Day weekend, Mastercon, a local hobby club that Chris was a member in, had a four-day event of workshops, get-togethers, contests, and an awards dinner. Chris looked forward to this every year to see his friends, share techniques and strategies about the craft, and be one of the judges in the contest. He loved seeing the different models. After what he had just been through, he needed some fun. While he spent time with his friends, Chris encouraged me to go on a bike ride. I thought it was a good idea and hoped I could work out those emotions I had been carrying inside me.

I went to the park where Chris and I went on our first bike ride together. It was a beautiful, warm, sunny morning – perfect for a ride. I warmed up to loosen my muscles then went right into a workout, pushing myself with sprints between the telephone poles. I was getting into a momentum when the vibration of my cell phone in my back jersey pocket disrupted my concentration, causing me to almost lose my footing on the pedals. I reached for my phone and saw it was Chris. Knowing I was on a bike ride, he wouldn't call unless it was an emergency.

"What's wrong?"

"Hi Steph. I'm okay. I'm starting to feel some pressure in my bladder again. I called Dr. Chehval and he told me to meet him at the emergency room."

"I'll be there as soon as I can." Hearing the panic in my voice, he tried to convince me that he was fine and to take my time. *Yeah, right!* I turned my bike around and sprinted the entire way back to my car which was about two miles away. Since I was still a new cyclist, this was a challenge, but I kept pedaling as fast as I could, hoping Chris was telling me the truth and was not in any pain.

When I got to the E.R., I was taken to the room where Chris was laying on a gurney, focusing on the ceiling.

"Hi babe," he said, smiling. "How was your bike ride?"

"It was fine," I answered, shocked, "but I think the most important question here is, how are *you* doing?"

"I'm hanging in there, but the pressure is starting to build up." Just then, a nurse came in with the supplies to flush the catheter. He made several attempts but the catheter was really blocked. Seeing Chris was becoming more uncomfortable, he called for Dr. Chehval and found out he was just finishing up with a patient. I held Chris' hand, but his body was so tense from the pressure, it was all he could do to just breathe. When Dr. Chehval finally came, he noticed the tension in Chris and helped him right away.

"Oh, thank you," Chris sighed with relief.

Dr. Chehval deflated the balloon in the bladder and took out a long, thin tube. This was the first time I was able to see the incision just below Chris' belly button. I finally understood what was going on with him. I studied my husband, feeling more amazed at how well he had been coping with all of this.

Dr. Chehval decided to increase the size of the tube, hoping it would take care of the problem. I asked what caused the blockage and he explained that sometimes calcium phosphate gets released in the urine and can get stuck in the tube.

"Unfortunately, it's one of the disadvantages of wearing a catheter," he said, "but it can be resolved by using a bigger sized tube."

After Dr. Chehval left the room, Chris turned to me, embarrassed. "I'm sorry you had to see this," he said, hiding his eyes. "I hope it didn't gross you out."

"What?! Chris, you're my husband and I'm your wife. What you're going through here, you are *not* alone. Look at me. I'm right here with you. Remember our vows: 'for better, for worse, in sickness, and in health?' I married you because I love you. I'm not grossed out. Instead, I'm amazed by your strength and optimism to keep going. I'm so proud of you," I choked.

Chris blinked several times. "Thanks, Steph. I love you too and I'm so lucky you're in my life."

"Oh Chris, we're both lucky."

We weren't just lucky, we were blessed. God gave us a special gift of love that most people search their whole lives for. When we found it together, we began to discover God's love within our love. For it says,

"Love one another for love comes from God. Everyone who loves is born of God and knows God. This is love: not that we have loved God, but that He first loved us and sent His Son as an atoning sacrifice for our sins. We have known the love of God and have believed in it. God is love. He who lives in love, lives in God and God in him."

- 1st John 4:7, 10, 16

When we left the ER, Chris checked his watch.

"Yep, I'll make it just in time to begin judging the models."

Stunned, I stared at him as he kissed me goodbye with a goofy grin. We finally made it around that pothole and we were riding on again.

Road Block

"Show me the way I should go."

- Psalm 143:8

A couple of days after Labor Day, I came home from school and found Chris downstairs working on one of his models. When I gave him a hug, I could tell something was wrong in the way he held me tightly. I felt that familiar pang in my chest.

"I have to tell you something," Chris said, letting me go. I pulled up a stool to sit in front of him. There was a stillness in the room when he took a deep breath and breathed out slowly, looking intensely into my eyes.

"Steph, I found another lump."

I froze, looking at my husband.

"Wh... what?" We stared at each other as I processed what he said. I held him tightly in my arms and felt tiny droplets on my shoulder. I fought back the tears knowing he needed me to be the strong one. I prayed for the words of hope we needed at that moment. I straightened myself in front of him and took charge.

"Okay, let's talk about this. Maybe it's scar tissue? You've been having a lot of problems with it and Dr. Hoffman wasn't able to remove any of it," I suggested.

"That makes sense," Chris nodded. We agreed not to jump to any conclusions and hoped for the best, rather than think of the worst.

"Did you call Dr. Chehval yet," I asked and found out that he scheduled a biopsy on Friday.

"It's going to be alright, Chris."

"Thank you for helping me through this," he whispered. I kissed his cheek and held him for a long time. When we separated, he was smiling.

The next day, I went to bed early while Chris stayed up to work on his model. Around 10:30, he shook me awake.

"Steph, we have to go to the emergency room," he said loudly.

I jumped out of bed. "What?" I asked, putting my hearing aids on. "What's wrong? Are you in pain?" Chris put his hands on my shoulders to calm me down.

"I'm okay, but I'm starting to feel some pressure in my bladder and I want to get to the E.R. before it gets worse."

"Let's go," I shouted but he stopped me.

"You might want to change first," he laughed. "I can wait a couple of minutes." I threw on jeans and a T-shirt, brushed my hair, grabbed my purse and keys and headed out to the garage where Chris was already in the passenger seat of my car. I gripped the steering wheel while my heart raced. Fortunately, it was late and the traffic was light on the highway.

"I'm okay, Steph," he repeated, patting my hand. "Take your time."

I drove to the entrance so Chris didn't have to walk very far and then parked in the closest spot. He was handing over the paperwork to the nurse when I ran in through the doors. I helped him sit in a chair and watched him lean back and close his eyes. I was amazed how he could be so calm while I kept checking the time, jiggling my leg, wondering how long it would be. Fortunately we didn't have to wait when someone called out Chris' name and we were led into a room where the nurse checked his vitals and recorded the problem he was having in the computer. We were taken to a room and were told that another nurse would be in shortly.

Chris undressed and sat on the gurney. Then we waited again. I didn't know how much time had passed and Chris started grunting. I looked around the room to see if there was a button to call someone for help when a nurse walked into the room. My shoulders dropped when I saw it was the same person who couldn't flush the catheter tube the last time we were here. I quickly told him it was the same problem as the previous week and explained how to relieve the pressure.

"Okay, let's take a look here," he said, examining Chris. After a few minutes, he told us that he would need to flush the catheter. I looked at him, baffled. *Why don't people ever listen to a husband's wife?* The nurse promised to be right back when he left to get the supplies he needed.

"Please hurry," I begged. We had to wait again and Chris was starting to feel more miserable, moaning louder. I looked around the room again to find the call button when the nurse returned. He worked to relieve the pressure, but nothing happened. He tried again and nothing. He started the process over and still no relief. Each attempt was causing Chris more pain and anguish. He apologized and told us that he would need to get a doctor.

"Hurry!" Chris yelled, grabbing the sheets on the gurney, leaning his head back.

I tried to help Chris relax by massaging his eyebrows, it wasn't helping him. I stroked his hand, but he pushed me away and grunted louder. I looked around the room for the call button, hoping it would somehow bring the nurse back in, but no one came. I rushed to the door, yanked it open and looked around. The place was deserted. *Where is everybody? I thought this was an emergency room that's supposed to be busy with doctors, nurses, and security.* Chris screamed again and I ran over to him. I looked at the catheter tube and wondered what I could do to take the damn thing out of him. Feeling clueless, helpless, and lost on how to help my husband. I flew over to the door again.

"Help Me! Somebody, please help my husband," I shouted, while Chris continued screaming in agony. I turned around to see him tearing at the sheets and shaking his shoulders in pain. I kept yelling for help until finally a doctor and the same nurse walked into the room.

"Okay folks, let's try to stay calm in here," the doctor said. Bewildered, I shook my head and folded my arms across my chest, fighting an incredible urge to smack her.

Please, doctor," I begged, "the pressure from the catheter is building up in the bladder and my husband is in so much pain." I couldn't see what she did to relieve Chris while I fought back the tears and tried to control the trembling in my body.

"Oh... thank you," Chris sighed. I turned around and saw his body relaxing as the urine flowed out of the opening below his belly button. I lost whatever control I had left and my body shook with such anger at how much my husband had to suffer just to get relief. I didn't know who to lash out against – the nurse who couldn't help, the doctor who took so long to come and her sarcasm, or Dr. Hoffman for doing this to my husband in the first place.

"Who is your doctor?" she asked interrupting my thoughts. I told her Dr. Chehval was Chris' doctor. She would call him to find out what he would want her to do and left the room. The nurse started caring for Chris while I tried to control the trembling in my body and fought back the tears. I couldn't speak. I couldn't move. I couldn't swallow the lump in my throat. I just stood there, struggling for sanity.

After awhile, Chris raised his hand for me to come by his side. I hadn't realized I was several feet away from him. I quickly wiped my eyes and went over to his side.

"I'm so sorry you had to see all of that." I shook my head.

"Huh? Oh, no, no, no. Chris, I'm so sorry you had to go through all of this." I fought the tears again, "I'm so very sorry." The nurse came back with the supplies to reinsert the tube and inflate the balloon that was still in the bladder. He told us that Dr. Chehval recommended staying with the same size tube and he would check it over during the biopsy in the morning.

It was around 1:30 in the morning, when we walked out of the E.R. Chris wanted to drive home and I started to argue.

"I'm too tired to talk about it," he said, holding his hand out for my keys. I climbed in the car, leaned back on the headrest and closed my eyes. I asked God to forgive my anger and frustrations, feeling ashamed. I checked on Chris. He caught my eye and winked. I thanked God that he was okay and we were able to go home together.

"When I said, 'My foot is slipping,' your love – oh Lord – supported me. When I was upset and beside myself, You calmed me down and cheered me up."

- Psalm 94:18 – 19

I closed my eyes and prayed again. *I can't do this without you, Lord. Please give me the kind of strength Chris needs from me to be there for him.*

I don't remember what we talked about or how it happened, but by the time we got home, Chris and I were laughing so hard, our stomachs hurt. We went straight to bed without changing our clothes and quickly fell asleep only to be jarred awake a few hours later by the screaming alarm clock.

When Dr. Chehval came in the pre-op holding area to see us, Chris told him about the difficulties he had with the catheter and how long it took for anyone to help him in the E.R. He apologized about how hard it was for us and promised to look into it. He went on to review the procedure with us.

"I will biopsy the nodule and send it over to the lab. I'll try to remove the scar tissue in the urethra and reinsert a catheter through it." He explained that he would clamp the suprapubic catheter and use it as a back up if there were any more problems.

"Okay, Doctor. Let's do it," Chris said, optimistically.

After watching Chris disappear into the operating room again, I met up with Teddie Momma in the waiting room. After my last experience of waiting, I knew I couldn't be by myself whenever Chris was in surgery. I received word that Dr. Chehval had begun the procedure. Teddie and I prayed and kept each other company. It wasn't very long when Dr. Chehval walked in the waiting room. I stood up and went off to the side with him. He told me Chris did well and was in the recovery room.

"The scar tissue was blocking about ten percent of the urethra which is about a fourth inch wide. I've tried several times to remove it, but it was too difficult to get through. I kept the suprapubic catheter in place and inserted a tube that is a size bigger. I hope this will resolve the blockage problems. Since Chris still has an opening at the perineum from the surgery last December, I inserted another catheter tube there as a back-up."

I looked down, trying to grasp how Chris would deal with two catheter tubes in two different places in his body. As if reading my mind, Dr. Chehval continued.

"This second catheter is only temporary to see how the larger sized tube works. This is the best we can do right now under the circumstances since there is another nodule we have to deal with. We'll find out what it is for sure in several days. In the meantime, I want Chris to get another PET scan. Hang in there and I'll be in touch next week," he said, patting my shoulder.

"Thank you, Doctor." I turned around and walked back to Teddie Momma, trying to remember to breathe. I sat down and she put her arm around me as I shared the information about the nodule.

"Steph, remember, *'God has not given you a spirit of fear, but a spirit of power, love, and a sound mind.'* God is in control. He is all over this thing for Chris." I let the scripture and her encouraging words settle into my mind and heart.

"I believe, Teddie. I know God is taking care of Chris. I will not give up." We prayed together and she stayed with me until I was called to join Chris.

"Thank you for helping me through this," I said and hugged Teddie goodbye.

Walking to Chris' room, I felt the strength build within my spirit. I knew God would give me the words to say to him to keep his faith strong.

"Hi. How are you feeling?"

"Okay," he mumbled. I walked over to his side.

"Did Dr. Chehval talk to you?" He nodded.

"Okay, what did he tell you?" Chris shared the same information I already heard and I could hear the frustration in his voice. I sat on the bed and positioned myself so he could see me.

"Chris, remember the scripture – God gave us a spirit of power (I pointed to my heart), of love (I leaned over and kissed him), and of a sound mind (I pointed to my head). He will give us the strength (I held his hand firmly) that we need to get through this while we put our faith in Him. We have God on our side."

I waited for Chris to think about it.

"Thanks, Steph. I needed to hear that," he said, smiling.

Writing this, I spent a lot of time reflecting and praying over this scripture from Second Timothy 1:7. If you run into a roadblock, don't let it stop you from pursuing on. Take a moment to remember that God gave you a spirit of power which comes from the Word of God. Read it, learn from it, and ride on with it. He gave you a spirit of love – to feel His love and to love each other through your race. He gave you a sound mind so that you can be at peace knowing God will do amazing things for you beyond anything you could hope for. Who better to fight for you than God? Use God's Word to get around that roadblock and to ride on strong in your race, no matter what happens.

It was as if we were put to the test on how we would handle the next roadblock we didn't see up ahead. Would we stop pedaling or keep on going, looking to God for His strength. During the second week of September, I came home and found Chris in his hobby room.

"Hi Chris," I hugged him and looked on his workbench. "How's your project coming along?" He turned me around and hugged me again.

"I'm glad you're home. I've been waiting all afternoon to talk to you." I started to sit down on the stool, but he took my hand and led me upstairs into the living room. I couldn't tell if he had good news or bad news.

"Chris, what's going on?"

"I had some problems with the catheter again so I went in to Dr. Chehval to get it taken care of," he told me calmly.

"Are you okay?"

"I'm better. Listen Steph, Dr. Chehval told me the results of the biopsy." I held my breath, hoping it was good news. "It's cancer – not scar tissue – and the PET scan showed cancerous activity in the prostate." Dumbfounded, I sat there looking at my husband in disbelief about what I had just heard.

"Cancer?" I whispered. Chris slowly nodded. *Oh my God. Another tumor!* "Chris, are you okay?"

"I'm fine now. How about you? How are you handling this?"

"I'm shocked."

"I was too, Steph, and angry. But I've had all afternoon to process it."

"What do we do now, Chris? What's the next step?

"We are going to keep on fighting. This cancer is not getting the best of me, Steph. We have a meeting with Dr. Chehval on Monday afternoon to go over everything and discuss my options. He and Dr. Needles suggest that I think about going to a cancer center in New York or to the one in Houston for another opinion. I'm thinking I should, but what do you think?"

"I think so. I'll do some research about both cancer centers and we'll brainstorm questions for Dr. Chehval. Let's just take things one day at a time and pray for guidance. How does that sound to you?"

"Thanks, babe, I really don't think I could get through this without you."

"We'll get through this and God will show us what to do."

"Let us approach the throne of grace with confidence, so that we may receive mercy and find help in our time of need."

- Hebrews 4:16

I looked at the date and noticed that it was almost exactly a year ago when we first learned about the cancer and we were back to where we first started. I shook my head, realizing that we still have a tough fight ahead of us. I had no idea just how hard it was going to be, but I knew we would be strong together through it. If Chris noticed the date, he never said anything about it and I didn't mention it to him.

While we waited for Dr. Chehval in his office, I wondered if I would ever get used to meeting him like this. He walked in quickly, shook our hands, and sat down at his desk. Chris didn't waste any time.

"Doctor, when you told me there was activity in the prostate, what does that mean, exactly?" Chris asked.

"It means there is cancer cell activity in the prostate, but *no* tumors," Dr. Chehval answered. "The good news is there is no sign of cancer in the urinary tract, bladder, kidneys, or in the lymph nodes."

"Chris didn't get to do all three courses of the first chemo treatment, is it possible to try it again?" I asked. Dr. Chehval looked in Chris' file.

"When you did the chemo last year, the tumor still grew."

"What about trying the cryosurgical technique again?" Chris asked.

"It has proven to work on these tumors. However we would still have to find a way to treat the cancerous activity in the prostate. Cryosurgery doesn't solve the problem since another tumor metastasized."

Dr. Chehval went on to tell us that he and Dr. Needles brought Chris' case back up at the team meeting and they reviewed everything we had done over the past year to brainstorm other options to treat this cancer. Since the first chemotherapy hadn't been very effective and surgery didn't stop the cancer, they discussed the possibility of radiation, however, it would be too difficult and painful for Chris to endure so radiation wasn't a valid option. The team suggested an aggressive surgical approach to treat this cancer: a penectomy (a partial or complete removal of the penis) and a cystoprostatectomy (the removal of the prostate and the bladder).

Chris was quiet and I held his hand. I took charge.

"But Doctor, why would it be necessary to remove the bladder if there is no sign of cancer in it? Why remove something when it's still healthy?" Before Dr. Chehval could answer me, Chris interrupted.

"What would you do if it were you, Doctor?

"Chris, if it was me," he paused, "I'd agree with the penectomy and remove the prostate. But before you decide on this kind of surgery, I strongly recommend that you get another opinion." Dr. Chehval waited patiently as we processed everything.

"Okay, I want to go to the cancer center in Houston," Chris blurted out. "What do we need to do?" Dr. Chehval called Sarah into his office to help us and suddenly everything was happening at a fast pace. I sat in Dr. Chehval's chair to use his phone to contact the cancer center, Chris called his insurance company to make sure he was eligible for services from there, and Sarah was organizing Chris' file for us. In less than an hour, we found out that we could use Chris' insurance and I had a contact person with a fax number to forward specific reports: diagnosis, chemotherapy treatments, surgeries, pathology and radiology reports, and a copy of the health insurance card. Later that afternoon, Sarah was able to fax all of the information successfully. All that was left to do was wait and pray.

Several days later, we had an appointment with Dr. Johnson during the first week of October.

"This is a good sign, Steph," he smiled. "I have a really good feeling about this doctor." *Oh God, I hope so.* I prayed that we chose the right path in our race and this doctor would be able to find a treatment protocol to cure my husband.

"I have put my trust in you. Show me the way I should go, for to you, I lift up my soul."

- Psalm 143:8

It was hard enough to hear the news that Chris still had cancer, but it was almost unbearable to have to tell our families and friends. Chris was very calm and confidant when he told the news to his brothers on the phone, assuring them he was going to beat it. But when the time came to tell Bob and Kelly, Chris really struggled to get the words out.

We went to their house for dinner several days after we met with Dr. Chehval. Throughout the meal, Chris kept the conversation away from cancer until he finally had the courage to bring it up.

"Bob, Kelly, there's no easy way to say this," Chris sighed. "The cancer came back." The only sound that could be heard was their kids playing downstairs as they looked at us with shocked expressions. Bob leaned forward, pressed his lips together and clenched his jaws tightly while Kelly stared at me with wide eyes.

"Guys, I have cancer, but it doesn't have me," Chris said and then told them about our plans to go to Houston. "I'm going to beat it."

After several minutes, Bob piped up.

"I know you will, buddy," Bob nodded. "If anyone can beat this thing, you can. And anything we can do to help you, we're here for you." Then he looked at me, "We're here for the both of you."

"We'll keep praying for you every day," Kelly promised.

Chris sat up taller as if he had received an extra dose of strength and energy from them. I realized at that moment, there was a special bond that only very close friends could experience and I felt overwhelmed by their love for us.

"A [true] friend will love you at all times and is closer to you than a relative."

- Proverbs 17:17 and 18:24

141

Angel's Wings

I truly believe that angels sometimes drift into one's life unexpectedly and just as suddenly, disappear before having the chance to thank them. That is when you realize the significance of their presence – to share God's love for you.

There was so much to do to prepare for our trip. Chris took charge of taking care of the dogs and the travel plans, while I concentrated on my job and organized my lesson plans for Teddie Momma, who agreed to be my sub. Through all of this, Chris was still having issues with the catheter and had to return to Dr. Chehval again. He taught Chris how to flush the catheter tube to relieve the pressure and gave him the supplies he needed. This was when Chris started taking care of the problems himself rather than going to the office all the time or to the E.R.

When we found out the cost of the airline tickets, hotel, rental car, meals, and the co-pays for the office visits, we were beginning to feel the financial burden since we had just paid off our wedding and honeymoon expenses. Someone told us about Corporate Angel Network – an organization that arranges transportation for cancer patients and their caregivers to and from cancer centers at no charge. After taking our information, we qualified for their services and they would be able to fly us to Houston. Within a couple of hours, everything was taken care of for us.

"Your Father knows what you need even before you ask Him."

- Matthew 6:8

When we arrived at the airport, we were told that we would be flying in a Falcon 2000 airplane. Two other people would be flying with us to Virginia and then we would go to Boston to transfer to another plane that would take us to Houston. Chris was so excited to be traveling in the type of aircraft that Michael flew in his job, he called Michael to tell him about it.

When we walked outside to the plane, the co-pilot greeted us and took our bags and a flight attendant took us to our seats. Once we boarded the plane, it was as if we stepped into a world of luxury. The panels were in a dark, rich shade of wood with a thin gold trim outlining the cabinets and windows. There were eight soft, beige leather recliners, two rows of two seats side by side, and toward the back of the plane there were two more seats at a polished, square table where we were asked to sit. After we sat down, Chris winked at me, leaned his head back and closed his eyes.

"Are you doing okay?" I asked, wondering how he was feeling.

"I'm doing great," he smiled. Relieved, I took a deep breath and started to relax. Chris pointed out a long, black limo pulling up near the plane and we saw an older gentleman who appeared to be in excellent physical shape easily climb out of the car.

"I can't believe it, Steph. I think that man was one of the admirals I served under while I was in the Navy."

We watched him walk next to a lady from the car to the plane. Chris leaned forward and whispered excitedly, "Yes, I'm almost positive that's him." We tried not to stare when they boarded the plane. I knew Chris would have loved to talk to him to find out, but we were asked to respect the two board members' space.

After take off, the flight attendant took our drink orders and brought us our lunch. We were served grilled boneless, skinless chicken breasts with fresh steamed vegetables and real mashed potatoes and gravy arranged artistically on real plates with gold-tinted utensils. Afterwards, we were given a choice of desserts. Chris opted for a slice of cheesecake and I chose chocolate cake with a cup of freshly brewed coffee. While we were winding down and settling in for the reminder of the flight, our fellow passengers walked to the back of the plane.

"May we join you?" the man asked and Chris excitedly answered *yes*. They sat on the couch across from us and we found out the gentleman was the admiral Chris served under during one of his tours. I noticed he sat up straighter during their conversation as they recalled some of the events that occurred. We also learned that the lady was a cancer survivor. She shared her story with us and encouraged Chris to keep fighting and not give up. She held my hand and told me to stay strong for my husband and advised me to take care of myself too. Chris told her how much we truly believed we would beat this.

"Yes," she slowly responded, studying him, "I believe you will."

We were interrupted by the pilot warning us that some slight turbulence was ahead, so they returned to their seats and buckled back in. With wide eyes and mouth agape, I looked at Chris who raised his hands, smiling.

"Only God," he whispered.

After we landed in Virginia, the passengers shook our hands and wished us well.

When we arrived in Boston, we were greeted by the flight attendant who took us to another Falcon jet. We started to move to the back of the aircraft and she invited us to sit in the front, explaining we were the only passengers on the flight. We were so surprised that they were waiting for us. We were not the owners or the partners or members of a board, but they were helping us in our journey to fight cancer. After we took off, we were served an assortment of fruit, cheese, crackers, chocolates, and gourmet cookies. Later, one of the pilots came back and spent some time with us. I leaned back on the headrest and watched my husband enjoy the conversation with him, learning as much as he could about the aircraft.

All the people behind the scenes and in both flights took the time to make sure we were taken care of and comfortable. I don't know how any of this happened, but I believed God's hand was in it, holding us in His palm as we soared through the skies with His angels.

After traveling all day, we had a free day to explore the cancer center. We took the hotel's shuttle to the medical office building where our appointment would be and discovered that the center was its own little city with buildings overshadowing block after block. We passed several medical buildings, a children's hospital, a regular hospital, and dormitories. Our building was seven floors high with long corridors about the length of a football field. The place was scrambling with so many people of all ages and from different ethnic backgrounds. But what affected us the most was seeing children fighting their own battle with cancer. At that point, Chris had had enough.

"Let's get back to the hotel and take a load off," he suggested.

I couldn't relax. I was already anxious to meet this new doctor. I reviewed our instructions, notes, and questions. I organized our backpack with our binder, an extra copy of Chris' medical file, his medical supplies, our snacks, a travel Scrabble game, a deck of cards, puzzle books, and magazines. Chris cleared his throat.

"Come over here and sit by me sweetheart," he said, imitating Humphrey Bogart, patting the empty space next to him on the bed. I laughed.

"Are you nervous?" I asked. Chris shook his head.

"No, just anxious like you," he answered, tickling me, making me laugh.

Just before I fell asleep in my husband's arm, I prayed again for God's guidance.

"'I will instruct you and teach you in the way you should go. I will counsel you and watch over you,' says the Lord."

- Psalm 32:8

We arrived a half-an-hour early for our first appointment – the new patient registration. But we still had to wait for our scheduled time. When it was our turn, the receptionist put a wide band on Chris' wrist that showed his full name, birth date, and his doctor with a barcode. He would have to keep it on the whole time we were there. After everything was entered in the computer, we headed up to the seventh floor for our appointment with Dr. Johnson. Up to this point, Chris had been doing well, but was starting to feel irritated with the catheter from the perineum. I kept him busy with a game of Scrabble while we waited for more than two hours until we were finally called in to see the doctor. We were taken into one of the patient rooms where the nurse checked and recorded Chris' vitals and asked a series of basic questions. We were told that Dr. Johnson would be in shortly and we waited again. My heart started pumping fast and I began to jiggle my leg, but Chris leaned back in his chair and closed his eyes. I opened our binder to the page with our notes and questions and started tapping my pen. Chris squeezed my hand.

"It's going to be okay," he said, smiling confidently.

The door opened and a tall, stocky man with tight, curly black hair walked in the room, followed by the nurse we met earlier. He introduced himself as Dr. Johnson and shook our hands when we told him our names. He sat down on the stool in front of us.

"I received a copy of your medical file and I'm aware of your case, and if you don't mind I would like to hear your story." Chris recounted everything while the nurse wrote notes in his chart.

"You have a rare cancer with very aggressive tumors that is difficult to treat and to cure, as you already know," Dr. Johnson began. "However, we do have an advantage that the cancer remains localized even though there is cell activity in the prostate. We need to get this thing under control so it doesn't spread into the lymph nodes or to a vital organ, then it would be incurable."

Gripping my pen, I froze. *"Incurable?"* I thought.

Chris squeezed my hand again.

"Doctor, have you had any experience treating this type of cancer?" Chris asked.

"I've had several patients and I am currently working with one with the same diagnosis," he said. Then he went on to share an idea of a chemo treatment he was considering for us to try with three different potent drugs: Taxol, Ifosfamide, and Cisplatin. But he wanted a few more tests to get a better idea of the cancer in Chris' body before making a decision on what to do next. The blood work was already scheduled followed by a chest X-ray after this meeting. We would have to return the next night for the MRI and come back in five days to find out the results.

God, are we doing the right thing here? Guide us in the direction you want us to go. I don't know what to do, but I do know I want what's best for my husband. You know what to do, please show us the way.

By the next morning, Chris was so irritated with the back-up catheter, he called Dr. Chehval. He talked Chris through the process of removing it. Afterwards, Chris was able to sit, lie down, and walk comfortably, but he was really sore. We talked about our meeting with Dr. Johnson and wondered about the chemo drugs. Chris hoped to do the treatments at home with Dr. Needles and I wanted to know about the side effects and how I could take care of my husband. In the meantime, we couldn't wait to see the doctor again. It was extremely difficult to wait being away from home, without our normal surroundings and routine. There were only so many Scrabble games we could play and movies to watch. When we found out Michael was driving down from his home in Dallas to be with us, Chris was so excited. He kept checking his watch and figuring out how much longer until he'd see his brother again. We were in the hotel lobby when Chris spotted Michael walking through the entrance and jumped out of his chair to meet him. Watching them embrace, I felt goose bumps all over seeing the joy and love between them. Even though distance separated them, the love between the four brothers stayed strong.

"He who loves his brother remains in the light and nothing in him will make him fall."

- 1st John 2:10

The Next Leg of the Race

Either you're coasting along in the wind and you're enjoying the ride from its strength or it's against you – challenging you to push through it or daring you to quit.

I wondered what would be ahead of us on this road we were riding on. Would there be more curves or would it be a straight, flat stretch? Would there be potholes in our way? Would we coast down some sloping hills or have to climb several steep hills? Would we have to battle against the headwinds or enjoy the tailwind?

One thing I knew for sure was that we had each other and God was with us. We believed He was leading us in the direction He wanted us to go.

"Whether you turn to the right or to the left, your ear will hear a voice behind you saying, 'This is the way, walk in it!'"

- Isaiah 30:21

Michael went with us to our appointment with Dr. Johnson and he became our strong support to lean on. We discovered that Chris' blood work was fine and the chest X-ray was okay. The MRI showed a questionable mass in the perineum. The doctor told us it could be scar tissue from the surgery, but we would need to keep an eye on it.

"I've decided to try Taxol, Ifosfamide, and Cisplatin together in a treatment called 'TIP,'" Dr. Johnson said. "Because all three drugs are so potent, we will have to spread it out over a four day period, during which you would need to stay in the hospital. Then you will have three weeks off to recover. I recommend two courses and do another MRI. If this treatment shrinks the tumor and reduces the cell activity in the prostate, then we would do two more courses."

"Doctor, we live in Missouri, is it possible I could do the treatment there with my oncologist, Dr. Needles?" Chris asked.

"You can do the treatment at home, but if it's possible, I would like you to do the first course here so I can monitor you and make any changes to your treatment," Dr. Johnson suggested. "I will contact Dr. Needles, but you need to know that I've taken over your case and I'm your primary oncologist." Chris agreed and we were relieved he could do the chemo treatment at home.

147

We found out that all three chemo drugs shared the same short-term side effects: loss of appetite, thinning or loss of hair, fatigue, nausea, constipation, headaches, and possibly mouth sores. Chris' blood count may drop after receiving the treatment, and he might experience numbness in fingers or toes and ringing in the ears.

"Stephanie," Dr. Johnson focused on me, "as a caregiver, I need you to note when these side effects occur and be ready to take care of Chris if and when they do occur. The nurse will give you further instructions on what to do."

Chris agreed to do the chemo. Several hours later, we found out that Chris was scheduled to arrive at the hospital the next day and would begin treatment as soon as he was settled in his room.

Having Michael with us gave us more strength and positive energy to keep riding on. He shared his optimistic hope and prayer with us that this next chemo treatment would bring us to victory.

That night as I watched my husband fall asleep, I tried to imagine how this chemo treatment would affect him. It was beyond what I could comprehend and I turned to God, hoping we were doing the right thing and this treatment, as potent as it was going to be for Chris, would destroy the cancer in his body.

"Trust in the Lord with all your heart, not on your own understanding."

- Proverbs 3:5

Once we checked into the hospital, Chris got settled in his room and was anxious to begin the chemo. After the nurse inserted an I.V. and started the fluids, she reviewed how the treatment would be carried out. On the first day, Chris would get all three drugs. Then on the second and third day, Chris would get an hour of Ifosfamide.

It was overwhelming to comprehend how much poison could be injected into a human's body to destroy cancer cells, which also destroy the healthy cells. I looked at my husband who took such excellent care of his body and yet, was agreeing to destroy it in order to fight cancer. I knew he had already given it up to God to give him the physical, mental, and spiritual strength to endure and persevere through it.

Chris was just beginning the last part of the treatment when it was getting late and he told me to catch the last shuttle for the hotel to get some sleep. Reluctantly, I kissed him goodnight and I when stepped outside his door, the tears flowed freely down my cheeks. Michael had

148

already left to go back home, so I had no company. When I walked into our hotel room, there was a sense of loneliness that was heavy in my heart. I decided to keep one hearing aid on and my cell phone close. But it didn't calm me enough and I tossed and turned all night. Not having Chris next to me took away my comfort, my warmth, my peace. I needed to feel his presence and to hold his hand. I prayed for God's loving comfort to help me relax and sleep.

The next thing I knew, I felt the warm sunlight on my face. I threw off the covers, showered, dressed and left for the hospital with an overnight bag. I was going to find a way to stay with Chris. I couldn't go through another night like that again.

When I walked in the room, Chris was smiling and already eating breakfast.

"Hi babe. How was your night?" he asked.

"Different," I paused. "I missed you too much."

A nurse who was checking Chris' I.V. overheard us and told me I could stay with Chris. She showed me how the chair opened up into a twin-sized mattress for a caregiver to sleep on and where the sheets, blankets, and pillows were stored. I was so happy I almost hugged her.

Over the next two days, I stayed close to Chris while he endured more of the chemo and the medications to off-set the side effects. He experienced nausea and ringing in his ears, but overall was tolerating everything well. When Chris wasn't sleeping, we watched movies, played Scrabble, and talked. Chris was very optimistic throughout the treatment and the nurses fell in love with his personality and positive attitude.

By Friday, he was doing so well, he was discharged earlier than expected. We were given a list of some of the medications and directions to keep the side-effects under control. The nurse explained each medicine, the purpose for it, and the best time of the day to take it. I was beginning to feel overwhelmed, wondering if I'll remember everything, and she showed me that all the directions she was giving me were already written on Chris' chart.

When we left the hospital, Chris was in a great mood and anxious to get back home. We spent the rest of the day making travel plans for Saturday and packed our suitcases and bags. Chris was beginning to show some signs of fatigue, so I did as much as I could for him without him realizing it – which wasn't an easy task since he was used to being so independent. Before we could leave, Chris had to report back to the cancer center first thing in the morning to get a Neulasta shot to help replace the white blood cells that were destroyed during the treatment.

We were able to use the services from the Corporate Angel Network again to fly home. Seeing that Chris had less energy than before and was getting easily tired, I was especially thankful for this wonderful organization to help us travel easily without the stress. He slept during the flight while I reviewed our instructions and wrote reminders to myself of the things I needed to take care of right away.

I wondered how Chris would be during the first week of rest after this chemo. Would his energy level get worse or improve? Would the ringing in his ears subside or increase? What other side effects would he have to deal with? Would he be okay at home while I worked? I felt the weight on my shoulders getting heavier as I pondered over these questions. I looked out the window and became lost in the clouds. I imagined we were flying through Heaven. Feeling as if we were as close to God as we could be, I prayed that this treatment would destroy the cancer in Chris' body and for the resilience he would need to deal with all of the side effects from it, and I asked for wisdom to help my husband in the way he needed me.

During the first week of rest, Chris slept a lot and didn't have much of an appetite. By the end of the week, the nausea and ringing in the ears had worn off and Chris' strength was slowly returning. One night, he climbed into bed with a silly grin.

"What's up?" I asked slowly and he pointed to the spot where his hair was thinning. He told me how he was washing his hair and saw clumps of it flowing down the drain.

"I'm gonna have fun with this," he said, pulling me close and kissing me. "Yeah baby, yeah," he laughed.

Mark came down to be with Chris during the second week of rest, and they went to Dr. Needles for a follow-up appointment to discuss the chemo regimen. I wasn't able to go with them because of the first quarter parent-teacher conferences and Chris promised to bring our binder with our notes for Dr. Needles. They talked about cutting out the third week of rest and start the second round only if the blood cell counts were stable. I didn't like this idea. I wanted Chris to have enough time to rebuild his strength to handle the second course of the chemo and the side effects. But he was getting back to his old self with a little more energy and he wanted to keep moving forward.

The next week, Chris went in for blood work and found out that all the numbers looked good and he could do the next round early. He would be admitted in the hospital on Halloween and stay four days. I wanted to be with him on the first day, but Chris insisted that I go to work and save my days for when he needed me the most. This was especially hard for me since I couldn't stay overnight with him at the hospital. I felt like I was in a constant tug-of-war between the responsibilities and demands of my job and the time I should be taking care of my husband. I also needed to take care of our three dogs, our home, and if I had any energy left, take care of myself too. All I could do was try to keep up and pray, pray, pray.

"True wisdom and strength belongs to God and comes from Him; [therefore] *we learn how to live and also what to live for through his counsel."*

- Job 12:13

While Chris was in the hospital, Dr. Needles checked on how he was handling the chemo each day. Dr. Chehval also stopped by to see Chris and changed the catheter tube for him.

"Steph, I still have very strong feelings about these two doctors," Chris told me one night at the hospital. "I feel that they genuinely care for me."

Chris tolerated the chemo regimen in the same manner as the first round and was discharged early on the fourth day. He had to return first thing on Monday morning for the Neulasta injection since the office wasn't open on the weekends.

This time, the side effects were harder on Chris. He was much more fatigued, the ringing was louder and more annoying, and his appetite was worse. By the end of the week, his hair was thinning so much that he gently washed his head until most of his hair was gone. When I came home from school, I was greeted by a pirate in my kitchen wearing a lime-green bandana and an eye patch.

"Arrr, I seemed to have lost me parrot," Chris exclaimed, looking around and then focused on me. "Arrr. Never mind. Come on over here, me lady, and I'll give you a kiss you'll never forget."

I put my book bag down, laughing at him and to my surprise he grabbed my waist, pulled me closer to him and gave me a kiss that I would never forget. Then Chris took off his bandanna and I kissed the top of his beautiful, bald, shining head.

"You're still sexy to me, babe."

A Blow Out!

"I cry to the Lord in a loud voice. My spirit grows faint, but You know my path."

- Psalm 142:1, 4

Chris' next appointment with Dr. Johnson was scheduled for mid-November. There were no available flights with the Corporate Angel Network. Chris didn't think he could handle the stress of traveling through the larger, busier airports, having to explain why he was wearing a catheter through the security checks, and sitting in the smaller seats on the plane. So we decided to drive. Poppa Bob offered to help us since it would be a long fourteen-hour trip and Chris gladly accepted it.

After a full day of traveling, we finally made it to our hotel and crashed in our rooms. Fortunately, we had time to get plenty of rest before the consultation appointment later in the afternoon with a new doctor, an urologist, to give us his opinion about the surgery.

I kept bouncing my knee while we waited for this doctor, anxious to know what he would tell us. There was a soft knock on the door and a short, thin man with black crew-cut hair in a white lab coat walked into the room and introduced himself as Dr. Fischer. He reviewed Chris' diagnosis and history of treatments and then asked to examine him. As I waited in the hallway, I wondered if Chris would ever get used to different doctors examining him, but he cooperated with dignity each time. When I came back into the room, I noticed the tension right away as Chris grabbed my hand tightly. *Oh God, give us strength.*

"You have a very complicated case," Dr. Fischer began. I felt the familiar tightness in my chest returning. "In my opinion, the first thing we need to do is to find the right kind of chemotherapy that will destroy the tumor and cancer cells. Once we get control of the cancer, then we would need to do a penectomy and remove the prostate." He paused. I felt like I was reliving the same nightmare and couldn't write down the words, gripping the pen, almost snapping it in half. I watched Dr. Fischer sit down on a stool across from Chris and looked compassionately at my husband.

152

"I'm sorry this is all very difficult to hear, but there is no other option in your case. We must control this cancer with chemo. It's pointless to do any kind of surgery if the chemo is not effective."

"Doctor, how long would it take to recover from this kind of surgery?" Chris asked.

"This would be a major surgery that could have you in the hospital between seven to ten days and then about six more weeks at home," Dr. Fischer answered.

"Have you had any experience with this type of surgery before?"

"Yes."

"What was the outcome?"

"They were successful," Dr. Fischer said optimistically.

"Would it be possible for reconstructive surgery afterwards?" Chris asked. We found out Chris would have to wait about two years to make sure the cancer was gone before doing reconstruction.

"What is important right now is to control the cancer," Dr. Fischer urged us. "I would like to do a cystoscopy of the pelvic area in order to develop a comprehensive plan for surgery after the chemo is successfully completed."

Chris slowly nodded, agreeing with the doctor. He told us the procedure was scheduled in five days. Dr. Fischer asked if we had any other questions, but neither of us could think of anything. He shook our hands and then walked out the door.

I kept blinking to keep the tears from escaping and gathered whatever strength I had left to pack our bag. I turned around slowly to face Chris. He stood there as if he was in shock. I dropped my bag and hugged him tightly. I wanted to tell him that it was all going to be okay, but I still couldn't find my voice.

"Let's get out of here," he said, taking my hand and led me out of the office.

When we returned to our hotel room, Chris needed to change the bandage around the suprapubic catheter and I called Poppa to talk about dinner plans. He didn't answer, so I went to his room and when he opened the door, I broke into sobs. He caught me and held me.

"I'm so sorry you two have to go through this. I wish I knew what I could do to help you," he said.

"You being here and praying for us is more than we could ever ask for right now, Poppa," I told him. I begged him not to let Chris or anyone else know what I've told him. But it helped that I had someone's shoulder to cry on for a little while. I felt completely spent as if I worked my body to the point of exhaustion. I prayed for strength to get through the next few hours and hoped that going out to dinner would be a good distraction for all of us. Poppa kept bringing up different topics to talk about during the meal, but nothing could get by Chris. He asked if I had told him about our appointment and Poppa said that he knew it was a tough meeting for us.

"Chris, I know you and Stephanie are going through a lot here and I wish I had the wisdom to shed some light on this. All you can do is take things one day at a time and hope for the best. And I'm here for you, any time – day or night."

It was as if this was what Chris needed to hear and he sat up taller.

"You're right. I'm not going to let this get the best of me."

"We are knocked down, but not crushed."

- 2nd Corinthians 4:9

"Jesus said, 'In this world you will continue to experience difficulties. But take heart, I have conquered the world.'"

- John 16:33

"No. In all of this we are more than conquerors, thanks to our Lord Jesus."

- Romans 8:37

Chris was already back on his bike and pedaling hard, refusing to give up.

The next morning we returned to the cancer center for blood work and an MRI. Since the MRI took about an hour, Poppa Bob and I decided to use the time to do some research in the cancer center's library. I tried to keep as much as I could private, but certain things weren't making sense to Poppa. I realized I could completely trust him and filled in the missing blanks on the details that no one else knew. At first he was stunned how much Chris had already been through in his fight. He helped me brainstorm ideas and shared some insights I hadn't thought of. I ended up with a full page of thoughts and questions to go over with Chris and the doctors. When we walked back to the MRI waiting room, I felt like I had a better handle on things and reminded myself that I can *"get through all things through Jesus, who gives me strength."* (Philippians 4:13)

Chris was all smiles when he walked out of the lab and clapped his hands.

"What do ya say we blow this joint and grab some lunch? I'm starving."

We had the rest of the weekend to ourselves so we decided to have a little fun and go sightseeing. After lunch, Chris and Poppa discovered an airplane museum not too far from us and they were as giddy as little boys oohing and aahing at the planes. They took their time checking out every part of each plane and reading the background information on it. I noticed they loved the older, propeller-driven planes as they stood next to each other with their eyes wide and heads tilted to the side, admiring them.

Since Chris was still feeling good, we decided to go to the Kennedy Space Center nearby where I became like a kid, exploring the museum. One of my favorite subjects to teach my fifth graders was Space. I couldn't wait to show them the pictures and tell them about the center. We had the opportunity to see the command center of the Apollo 11's landing on the moon mission. Everything was exactly in place as the tour guide shared details of the room. To top off our field trip, we walked the length of a Saturn V rocket that was laid out horizontally in a long, rectangular warehouse.

Saturday we took a road trip to Galveston to hang out at the beach. It was a beautiful, sunny day for November that made it exhilarating to enjoy the soft white sand and the warm ocean breeze. We listened to the waves softly slapping the shores and watched the sea gulls flying around us, calling to each other and searching for their dinner.

"It doesn't get any better than this," Poppa said, taking in the scenery.

Later, we went to see the Christmas lights display. We didn't know it was a walking tour and I was concerned it might be too much for Chris, but he convinced me he was having fun. There were thousands of lights streaming across and along our walking paths so that it became a world of imagination and color in the dark night. There were so many different displays on the tour, which ended with the Nativity Scene, brilliantly lit up, putting us in the Christmas spirit.

After two days of activities, we decided to take it easy and stayed at the hotel. I reviewed the research, notes, and questions with Chris, but he wasn't worried. He just wanted to know for sure if the chemo was effective since the tumor felt softer.

The appointments were running on schedule and we were called on time to meet with Dr. Johnson. We found out that the blood work was fine, but the MRI showed that the tumor hadn't shrunk as much as it should have with the type of chemo Chris endured.

What? The chemo wasn't effective? It felt like a ton of bricks landed right in the middle of my chest.

"There is a possibility of a tumor in the perineum that was originally speculated to be scar tissue," Dr. Johnson said. I shook my head in disbelief. *Two tumors? God, help us.* I couldn't bear to look at Chris.

"I have another idea," Dr. Johnson continued. "It is a chemo treatment called MVAC that consist of four very strong chemo drugs: Methotrexate, Vinblastine, Adriamycin, and Cisplatin. It has been used for bladder cancer, however it has never been tried for urethral cancer and it is not FDA approved for it. I know you've tried Cisplatin in the previous two regimens, but the other three were never tried against squamous cell tumors before. Since they are very strong, potent drugs it is a possibility that all four of them together would make an impact against this cancer."

We asked if the insurance company would agree to this treatment if it wasn't FDA approved and Dr. Johnson assured us that they would get approval for it.

"Let's do it," Chris said confidently. Dr. Johnson would contact Dr. Needles to start the treatment the following week at home. We met up with Poppa Bob and Chris told him what was going on.

"This treatment is going to work," Chris told us, smiling.

I looked at my husband, once again amazed at his strength, his confidence, and his faith. I remembered the scripture Teddie Momma often told me, as if I was hearing her voice, "Steph, God did not give you a spirit of fear, but of power, love, and a sound mind. Just have faith." Chris exemplified that power within his spirit.

The next afternoon, we returned for the cystoscopy and I prayed for some good news.

"Chris is doing well and is recovering. There are no signs of cancer in the bladder," Dr. Fischer said. "I have a better understanding of what's going on with him. But right now, we must find the right treatment protocol to control and treat this cancer before doing any kind of surgery." I prayed again for God's direction and guidance to find the right chemo to battle this cancer for us.

"I am the Lord, the God of all mankind. Is anything too hard for me?"

- Jeremiah 32:27

Chris recovered easily from the procedure and we were anxious to get home. We couldn't wait to celebrate our first Thanksgiving together as husband and wife and with my family.

It seemed like the trip took much longer even though we made fewer stops and Chris did most of the driving without any problems. Once we got home, he was so tired that he fell asleep on the couch. I offered to help him in bed, but he didn't want to move. Since the next day was a holiday, I had to go to the store to get a few things we needed before they closed. When I got home, Chris was where I left him, but looking very pale. I felt his forehead and it was burning hot. I took his temperature and saw he had a 102 degree fever. I wanted to call Dr. Needles, but Chris thought it was because he was really tired from the long drive. I shook my head, worried if he was coming down with an infection. A couple of hours later, I checked Chris' temperature and it went down one degree. Around four in the morning, Chris became restless and his temperature went back up to 102 degrees. I called the exchange number and talked to Dr. Needles. He suggested giving Chris Tylenol to see if it would bring the fever down. Several hours later, his temperature dropped to 99 degrees.

I wanted to stay home so he could rest, but he insisted on going to my sister's.

"Steph, I want to celebrate Thanksgiving with your family. Come on. I'll be okay, my temperature is steady. I'll even let you drive."

I knew it meant a lot to him, but I still had my doubts. On the way, Chris slouched in the passenger seat and rested his face against the window.

"Chris, are you okay?" He smiled and said that the coolness of the window felt good to him. *Uh-Oh, that's not good.* I wondered if his temperature went back up. When we arrived at Carol's, Chris admitted he was feeling worse and wanted to go back home. I took his temperature again and it was 103 degrees. I called Dr. Needles and he told me to get Chris to the E.R. Trying not to panic, I went inside to tell Carol what was going on and then rushed out the door, drying my eyes and doing my hardest to remain composed and strong for Chris. I prayed for God's protection over my husband.

"God is our strength and protection, an ever present help in trouble."

- Psalm 46:1

Once we got to the E.R., a nurse started an I.V. of fluids and antibiotics and a doctor ordered some tests: a chest x-ray – which showed his lungs to be clear and healthy, a urine culture, and a blood test. After several hours, Chris was taken to a room in the hospital and was still sleeping. I let the tears flow freely and hoped it would release the weight in my chest. I couldn't imagine what was wrong. I prayed again for God's healing over his body and from this cancer. I knew that nothing was impossible for Him to accomplish.

"Anyone who is having trouble(s) should pray!"

- James 5:13

After some time, I felt a gentle squeeze on my shoulder and looked up at Chris' nurse.

"Your husband will sleep through the rest of the night and I promise to check on him often. You've been through a lot today. You should go home and get some rest." I didn't want to leave Chris, but I knew she was right, already feeling sore and strained.

"Sleep well Chris. I'll see you first thing in the morning," I whispered in his ear and kissed his cheek.

When I walked in my house, I realized that our first Thanksgiving was over. Dumbfounded and completely spent, I sat at the table all alone, buried my head in my hands and let the tears flow.

I was thankful for the holiday break and I was able to spend a lot of time with Chris. By Sunday, he was back to his old self again and insisted that it was just a fluke. Bob, Kelly, and their kids came by for awhile and really cheered us up with their sense of humor and positive energy. After they left, Chris was in much better spirits.

Later that afternoon, an infectious disease specialist came by. I didn't know there was such a specialty.

"Chris, I'm sorry to tell you this in the middle of all that you're going through. The blood tests shows that you have a staph infection and you will need to be on a very strong antibiotic called Vancomycin to combat it. You won't be able to resume chemotherapy until it is cleared." It felt like someone punched me in the middle of my chest and knocked the wind out of me. I leaned back in the chair and slowly turned to Chris. The look on his face hit me harder than the news.

"Steph, don't start crying, please," he said firmly. "This is bad enough for me to handle right now and I can't deal with it if you start crying." It was the first time he has ever spoken to me like that. I blinked about a hundred times to stop the tears and took many deep breaths to drown the overwhelming emotions that were bottling up inside of me. I focused on the doctor.

"How did Chris get a staph infection as meticulous as he is taking care of himself and as I am to keep everything clean for him?" I asked. Because Chris' immune system was so low, he could have caught it from anywhere and from anyone.

That night, I rested my hand on Chris' pillow, wishing desperately he was here with me and the tears turned into sobs. I pleaded to God to rescue us from this blow out.

"My spirit grows faint, but You know my path. I cry out to You. You are my refuge. Listen to my cry, for I am in deep despair."

\- Psalm 142:4, 6, 7

After several days, the tests showed that Chris was responding well to the antibiotics and by the end of the week, he was released with a picc line – an IV catheter that was inserted into a deep, larger vein in his arm to continue the treatment at home. Chris adapted to it while he continued to do some of the chores around the house, cared for the dogs, and worked on his models. However, he had some frustrating moments with the limitations from the picc line as well as issues with the suprapubic catheter. Fortunately, he had a visiting nurse who came twice a week to check on him and to get blood work. She helped him get through those tough moments which gave him the strength to take things one day at a time.

Chris was finally cleared from the staph infection 27 days later and the nurse withdrew the picc line just before Christmas. I came home from school to find Chris strutting around the kitchen and swaying his arms with a wide grin on his face.

"Hi Steph. Notice anything different?" I jumped up excited, dropping my bags, and embraced my husband. He still had to continue the treatment with oral antibiotics for 12 more days, but I couldn't have asked for a better Christmas present for Chris and thanked God for healing him from this infection.

Rolling Hills

After finally getting over that steep hill, sometimes there are many smaller hills to climb in the journey before reaching a flat stretch.

Bob called Chris the *King of the Hills.*

"Chris' cycling abilities were one that was part cheetah and part bear – lightning fast, with strength and power. He never backed down from the challenge to reach the top, and he never gave up or got off his bike. He would climb steadily, pacing himself, and pushing his legs to keep pedaling. He would reach the top victoriously and if the hills were alive, they'd bow humbly to him.

Lazy and complacency were not in our vocabulary," Bob said. "We were very competitive and would never admit when we were in pain or hurt, because if one of us let the other know, he would turn up the heat and go. However, we would rather die than let the other one down during our rides. We would dig down deep within ourselves, let go of our ego and pride to encourage, motivate, and support each other. Riding together made us both better as a person and as a cyclist."

I believe Chris' mentality from cycling helped him endure so much and stay strong in his fight against the cancer. From January to mid-July, Chris experimented with eight more chemo drugs in four different regimens. He suffered from swelling in his feet, ankles, and legs, mouth sores, a rash and dry skin, constant urinary tract infections and bladder spasms, blockages from the catheter tube, and stabbing pains from the tumors. But he kept riding on.

By the end of April, Dr. Chehval and Chris discovered another nodule in the penis. We were in the middle of the fifth chemo regimen and now Chris had three tumors in the penis and one in the perineum.

"It's okay, Steph. We're going to find the right chemo. I have good doctors who won't give up. I have you by my side and I know God is helping us through this fight." Chris' faith and courage was astounding. It was as if he was telling me,

"But me, I'm not giving up. I'm sticking around to see what God will do. I'm waiting for God to make things right. I'm counting on God to listen to me. I'm down, but I'm not out. I'm sitting in the dark right now,

but God is my light. He's on my side and is going to get me out of this. He'll turn on the lights and show me His ways."

- Micah 7:7 – 9

Chris discovered what patience really entailed in his race. Like an athlete who sets deadlines for himself in his training, Chris was setting up recovery time from various treatments and surgical procedures, thinking he'd be back to doing normal activities and riding his bicycle again. However, he realized that he couldn't set those kinds of deadlines anymore and began to focus on doing the best he can, one day at a time. Chris wrote *"Everyday is a good day"* on Post-It notes and displayed them all over the house as a visual reminder – no matter what happened, it would be a good day. This helped us get through the next two months until we hit another hill.

We were in the middle of the sixth treatment, when I heard Chris yell out from our bathroom. I rushed to him from the living room.

"Chris?"

"Don't come in," he shouted. "I'm okay. I'll be out in a few minutes."

I didn't like how he sounded, so I waited in our bedroom. Those few minutes turned into a long half-hour when Chris finally opened the door, looking very pale with fear in his wide eyes.

"Chris, what happened?" He took my hand and led me into the living room. I noticed how he struggled to sit down, breathing slowly and deeply. *Oh God, something is really wrong.* I knew I had to be patient for him to tell me while I fought the panic rising in my chest.

"Steph, one of the tumors in the penis broke through the skin," he whispered.

My eyes widened and I held my breath, trying to comprehend what he was telling me. *What is happening to my husband? God, please help us.*

"I'm scared, Steph," he said, trembling. *So am I.*

"It's going to be okay Chris," I whispered. I immediately called Dr. Needles and he suggested putting an antibiotic ointment over the area.

Over the next week, the pain from all the tumors intensified and Chris felt more miserable. It had been 10 days since the chemo. I began to question if it worked at all, but I refused to think negatively and stayed hopeful. I called the exchange again for advice on how to relieve Chris' pain. The doctor on call increased the dose of the pain medicine and a few hours later, Chris finally found relief and slept the rest of the evening and through the night.

Feeling completely spent from seeing Chris in so much pain, I broke down and sobbed in the living room. Benji laid on my feet, Bridget cuddled close to me on the couch, and D'Artagnon sat in front of me – all looking at me with sad eyes as if they were saying, *"Oh mom, what can we do to make you happy again?"* Seeing their expression, I wondered if it was how I looked to Chris whenever he was hurting. The dogs stayed near me and I felt their love, which gave me comfort. I prayed and hoped Chris felt comforted by my presence and my love just as much.

The appointment with Dr. Needles in the beginning of July couldn't come soon enough. The CT-scan didn't show any new tumors other than the four and I breathed a sigh of relief.

"But," Dr. Needles paused. I sat up, rigid in my chair. "There is a questionable spot in the lower left lung." *Huh? Did I just hear him say there was a spot on Chris' lung?* I looked over at Chris who was frowning, listening to Dr. Needles.

"To be sure," he continued, "I want a CT-scan of the chest and an MRI of the pelvic area." *Oh God, help us through this.*

Neither of us said anything on the way home. When Chris parked the car in the garage, he unbuckled his seatbelt and sat still for a long time.

"You know what?" Chris shouted, making me jump. "I'm not going to count this appointment. I'll do the MRI and a CT-scan of my chest and we'll know for sure what's going on. I'm not letting this cancer get the best of me. I'm going to let this go and let God handle it. Okay?"

I stared at my husband in awe.

"I need to hear you say it, Steph."

"Okay, Chris," I nodded. "So, why are we still sitting in the car?"

"That's my girl," he laughed.

Feeling overwhelmed from the news, I felt a desperate need to be rescued. I didn't want to break down in front of Chris so I asked him to take the dogs outside while I took a shower. Once I turned on the hot water, I let go and my body rocked with sobs. I braced the walls for support and shivered. *Oh God, save me from these fears, because they mean death for Chris. I'm afraid, but I believe in Your Word, which is full of life. Save Chris from this cancer. Nothing is impossible for you, oh God. Show the doctors what to do for him. Tell me what to do and show me how to do it. I can't ride up this hill without You.*

After the shower, my body relaxed and I felt a sense of peace within me that I could not understand. I was strongly compelled to look through my Bible. I didn't know what I was searching for, so I re-read the passages I high-lighted and was led to Psalm 116. It wasn't marked, so I continued to thumb through the pages. The next thing I knew, I went back to it and noticed the words:

"You have freed me from death. Because He has not been deaf to me, I will call on Him as long as I live. When the cords of death entangled me, the snares of the grave laid hold of me, when affliction got the better of me, I called upon the Lord, 'Save my life!' Gracious and righteous is the Lord; full of compassion is our God. He has freed my soul from death, my eyes from weeping, my feet from stumbling; I will walk before the Lord in the land of the living."

Chris walked in the living room and was immediately concerned about me. I gave my Bible to him and explained how I was led to this particular psalm. He read the verses out loud.

"Wow," he whispered.

"What do you think it means, Chris?"

"I don't know, Steph." He looked at me with tears in his eyes, smiling. "But I believe God is telling us that I'm going to be healed from this cancer."

"We're going to keep believing, Chris, no matter what happens."

Over the next week, Chris struggled with sitting, lying in bed, and moving around due to the pain and discomfort from the tumors, especially from the one that had broken through. It felt like our faith was being tested, but we kept taking it one day at a time, without giving up hope.

During the appointment with Dr. Needles, he examined Chris and advised him to continue applying the antibiotic ointment on the tumor and keep it bandaged. When I came back into the room, he sat on the stool in front of us and let out a long sigh.

"The tumors have grown and the CT-scan showed four tiny spots in the lower lungs." Looking at Chris, he continued. "The CT-scan back in November didn't detect anything, so this is a new discovery."

I wrote "JESUS" in the middle of our notebook.

"Is it possible to do surgery to remove the tumors and the spots in my lungs?" Chris asked. Dr. Needles pressed his lips together and shook his head.

Stephanie M. Saulet

"If we were to do the surgery, it would be very aggressive. But it doesn't solve the problem – it won't cure the cancer since there are cancerous cells in your body. We have to find a chemo regimen that will work to get control over this cancer."

How many times have we heard this? God, what is the right treatment?

Dr. Needles wanted to brainstorm with Dr. Johnson on another idea he had in mind and rescheduled us to return the following week.

Another week of waiting? Oh Lord!

Chris was very quiet when we left the office and I worried about how this was affecting him. He put the key in the ignition and turned on the air conditioner, but kept the car in Park. Somehow I knew this was a crucial moment for us – would we stop or keep pedaling up this hill? I prayed for wisdom.

"Chris, I know the news was discouraging, but we are not giving up. God is working on healing you. Remember what you said about believing in our faith? Remember that psalm? Even though the doctors don't know what to do, God does. Let's pray for Him to guide Dr. Needles on what to do next. We're not alone with God on our side." I grabbed Chris' right hand and held it up. "He is holding us with His right hand, giving us the strength we need as He continues to fight for us. I don't know how or what or when, but I believe God *will* heal you."

Chris sat there for several minutes.

"Okay," he said, smiling, "I believe it too. I'm not giving up."

On the drive home, I remembered a scripture that we read early in our race:

"Fear not, for I am with you. Be not dismayed, for I am your God. I will strengthen you, yes, I will help you, I will uphold you with My righteous right hand and those who war against you shall be as nothing, as a nonexistent thing. For I, the Lord your God, will hold your right hand, saying to you, 'Fear not, I will help you!'"

- Isaiah 41:10 – 13

To get through the next week, we decided to decorate our kitchen and dining room. Chris did well painting and putting up the border without suffering much pain. However, the day before the appointment with Dr. Needles, Chris felt painful stabs from the tumor that broke through the skin that made him fall to his knees. After several long, agonizing minutes, I helped Chris up and walked him slowly to the couch. I called the office and was told to increase the pain medicine. A few hours later, Chris finally found relief and slept for the rest of the day and through the night. Watching over him, I cried silent tears seeing my husband in so much pain. I prayed again with hope for the right chemo treatment to heal Chris.

Back at the office, I wrote *JESUS* on a new page in our notebook to focus on during the meeting, believing I would feel His strength from His name. The door suddenly opened. Dr. Needles quickly walked in and sat on the stool in front of us.

"I spoke with Dr. Johnson for a long time. He suggested Avastin which works to inhibit the blood vessels to the tumors to prevent them from growing. But the insurance company won't approve it unless we can find a chemo drug that'll work first." Dr. Needles paused. "Dr. Johnson doesn't have any more ideas on what to try next." I held my breath and looked at *JESUS* on my paper.

"So, I looked into Oxaliplatin and have approval to try it. I suggest doing four courses once every two weeks. Then we'll do another MRI and go from there."

"Let's do it. When can I start?" Chris asked.

"Now," Dr. Needles said and handed the order to him.

When we walked into the treatment room for the seventh chemo regimen, Chris squeezed my hand, "Steph, this one is going to work."

"Be brave. Be strong. Don't give up. Expect God to get here soon."
- Psalm 31:24

The nurse told Chris that he would have to have a port after this round because Oxaliplatin was especially hard on the veins and caused painful sensations for the patient.

"No. I've handled the other chemo well, I can handle this one too," Chris said confidently. The nurse suggested taking one thing at a time and explained that the main side effect from this chemo was extreme sensitivity to cold. Chris would not be able to eat, drink, touch, or breathe in anything cold.

"Wait!" Chris cried out with wide eyes. I jumped, thinking something was wrong. "Does this mean I can't have Fritz's ice cream?" he asked seriously.

"No, I'm sorry, not while you're on this treatment," she said sympathetically.

"Well, okay. It'll be one more thing I have to look forward to when I beat this cancer," Chris said optimistically.

The nurse looked at me with wide eyes and whispered, "Wow."

She suggested Chris wear warm gloves and socks at all times to keep his fingers and toes warm. If he felt tightness in his throat after breathing in cool or cold air, he should cup his hands over his mouth to breath in his own warm air until it went away. This was going to be a challenge since we were in the middle of the summer with air conditioning.

After about five minutes into the treatment, Chris yelled, feeling painful sensations flow from his hand into his wrist and up his arm. The nurse injected something in his I.V. and he was relieved right away.

"Okay," he nodded breathlessly, "Okay, I want a port."

While Chris slept through the chemo, I prayed again that this one would work against the cancer, for God's supernatural healing in Chris' body and thanked Him for Dr. Needles who was still fighting for us.

"I will watch in hope for the Lord, my God will hear me."

– Micah 7:7

Four days after the chemo, Chris had the surgery to implant a venous access port in the right side of his chest. I felt so sad for him to have to deal with a port, the suprapubic catheter, and the pains from the tumors. For me – it would be too much – but for Chris – it was like that steep hill, challenging him to quit. He didn't let it get to him and he continued to dominate the hill.

When Chris woke up from the procedure, I asked if he was in any pain.

"Nope," he smiled, "it's all good," and gave me two thumbs up.

Overall, Chris experienced minimal side effects from the chemo and was tolerating the port well. The tumor in the perineum felt different and softer. We were all hopeful this regimen was working and Dr. Needles increased the dosage for the last two rounds. The pain was under control and Chris was able to sit and lay down comfortably.

Life was good again and we took advantage of it. We spent an afternoon at a park for a picnic and got together with some friends we hadn't seen in a long time. We finished decorating our kitchen and dining room. Chris continued to walk several miles a day on the treadmill, but he desperately missed riding his bike. He knew he had to be patient and kept looking ahead.

"By entering through faith into what God has always wanted to do for us, we have it all together with God because of Jesus. We should feel secure, even in our troubles because we know how troubles can develop passionate patience in us and how that patience in turn forges

the tempered steel of virtue, keeping us alert for whatever God will do next. Hope does not disappoint us because of the Holy Spirit which has been given to us to show us the love of God within our hearts."

- Romans 5:1, 3 – 5

Over Labor Day weekend, Chris started feeling stabbing pains from the tumor that broke through and the one in the perineum. This was not a good sign, but we refused to give up hope.

Waiting for Dr. Needles was still excruciating. I couldn't shake the anticipation of what he would tell us, jiggling my leg and tapping my pen against our notebook. I glanced at Chris, wondering how he was doing. His eyes were closed, his head tilted back against the wall, and his arms folded across his chest.

"Chris," I exclaimed, baffled, "how can you be so calm, sitting there?"

"Well, how do you expect me to sit in a chair?" he asked with a quizzical expression and winked. I started to answer him, but Dr. Needles walked in the room slowly. He opened Chris' file and studied his notes quietly. For the first time since our first meeting two years ago, I noticed how much thicker it had gotten and felt a sickening feeling in the pit of my stomach. After several long minutes, he finally faced us with a grim expression, resting his elbows on his knees, and leaned toward Chris.

"The tumor in the perineum did change shape," he paused, "but it grew from 5.8 to 7.2 centimeters. The other tumors grew a centimeter, making two of them about 5 centimeters and one about 2 centimeters." Neither of us could say anything even though our mouths were wide open.

"Chris, since the diagnosis, you have gone through 12 different chemo drugs in seven regimens – we've used Cisplatin in four of those," he paused again. "I admit that I'm frustrated, trying to figure out what chemo to try next." *Oh God, please don't let him give up on us.*

"Doc...," Chris cleared his throat and sat up straighter, "Dr. Needles, I want to keep on fighting."

"Okay," he said slowly. "I talked with the radiation oncologists and they are willing to try it. But Chris, it will be very invasive and the side effects will be extremely painful."

I felt a lump form in my throat and a huge knot in my stomach, making me feel nauseous. I couldn't write any more notes. Several long minutes passed and Chris nodded confidently.

"I'll get through it."

After Dr. Needles left the room, I was still glued to my seat. Chris took my hand and pulled me up to him, waking me from my shocked state.

"Steph, I'm not giving up. This cancer may think it's winning the battle, but I'm going to win the war. I know God will give me the strength and I know you will stay by my side through it."

After climbing so many hills, we found ourselves on a flat stretch without knowing where it would lead us. But we knew God was with us and would give us the strength to keep riding on in our race.

Fire

"When you walk through fire, you will not be burned; the flames will not consume you. For I am your Savior, I, Yahweh your God. You are precious in my sight – I have loved you. Fear not, I am with you."
- Isaiah 43:2, 3, 4, 5

Chris was geared up for this new leg of the race and anxious to start radiation as soon as possible. I wanted to know how we could be prepared for the side effects and I couldn't help worrying about how painful it might be for my husband.

Chris raised his arm for me to come by his side.

"Are you in pain?" I asked, concerned.

"No," he smiled and wrapped his arm around my waist. "No worries," he whispered in my ear and kissed my cheek. There was a soft knock on the door and a man with short, black hair in a white lab coat walked in, introducing himself as Dr. O'Brian and shook our hands. He went through an interview with Chris and asked to examine him. When I returned, he told us he was aware of Chris' case from Dr. Needles.

"Since chemo hasn't been effective against the tumors, radiation is the last resort to try to control this cancer," he said. "Chris, you need to understand it will be very invasive and painful since the tumors are so close under the skin." I struggled to breathe, wondering how much more pain Chris could take.

"If you agree to do this," Chris nodded and he continued. "You'll get radiation for 15 minutes Monday through Friday for six to seven weeks. We'll meet once each week to re-evaluate."

"Okay, how soon can I start?" Chris asked.

Dr. O'Brian told us the radiation technicians needed to map out the areas and tattoo the places for the radiation beams, create a block to cover the rest of Chris' body, and make a cradle for him to lie on during the treatments. Chris would be able to start the following week, which would be the third week of September.

"Let's do it," Chris said.

I couldn't be with Chris for his first radiation treatment because of an important event at school, but I called as soon as I could to find out how he was doing.

"It was like I had a 15 minute snooze," he said, laughing and I was relieved he was okay. Later that night, Chris noticed some swelling and I prayed again for the strength he would need to endure this.

Over the next two weeks, the swelling from the radiation gradually worsened, making it harder for Chris to sit or lie in bed comfortably. I explored different kinds of cushions, pillows, and chairs for him. Once we'd find a way, it would work for a few days and then he would feel uncomfortable again and we'd start over. Chris struggled the most at night when he needed sleep. Some nights we would find a way for him to lie in bed comfortably, but most nights, nothing worked and we'd struggled to try one thing after another. The lack of sleep made it hard for us to get through each day. So, we decided to deal with the day and the night separately. To our surprise, it made it easier for us to get through it all while still praying for strength and perseverance.

The beginning of the third week of radiation, Dr. Needles started Chris on Hydroxyurea – a chemo pill Dr. O'Brian suggested that could enhance the effectiveness of the radiation. Chris would have to have blood work every week to make sure he could continue the daily chemo. Two weeks later, which was the beginning of the fifth week of radiation, Dr. Needles increased the Hydroxyurea to twice a day and added Bleomycin to the regimen. We had been reluctant to try it because of how damaging it could be to the lungs, but felt we reached a point that we had no other choice.

Even though Chris and I had read and prayed over many scriptures, there was one we focused on during the radiation treatments:

"Don't be afraid: I'm with you. I've called your name. You are mine. When you're in over your head, I'll be there with you. When you're in rough waters, you will not go down. When you're between a rock and a hard place, it won't be a dead end – because I am God, your personal God, I paid a huge price for you. That's how much you mean to me! That's how much I love you! So, don't be afraid: I'm with you."

- Isaiah 43: 2 – 7

At the start of the sixth week, Chris reached a breaking point. Nothing worked to help him get comfortable and relax. The pain and the many restless nights wore him down. I took a morning off to be with Chris for his appointments with Dr. Needles and Dr. O'Brian. I found out Chris lost 14 pounds since starting radiation. Dr. Needles suggested taking a week off from radiation, re-adjusted the pain medication, and prescribed Ativan to help Chris' body to relax enough to sleep at night. Dr. O'Brian agreed and rescheduled Chris' treatment for the next week.

I returned to work in the afternoon and then picked up Chris' prescriptions on my way home. Throughout the drive, my mind wandered in many directions. I reviewed our meetings that morning. I thought about my first quarter conferences with my students' parents. I had a new idea to help Chris sit and lay down comfortably. I wondered what to make him for dinner to entice his appetite. Suddenly, I was crushed by an air bag.

I sat there trying to process what had just happened as the air bag deployed, smelling burnt rubber, and slowly I saw the damage in front of me. Realizing I was in a car accident, I immediately jumped out of my car and rushed to the vehicle in front of me and saw it was a young man either in his late teens or early 20's. He appeared to be stunned, but I didn't notice any injuries on him. Surveying the scene, I saw he had hit the SUV in front of him with a mother and a small child in the back seat. Watching her comfort her child, I couldn't move.

Looking around, I felt my breath catch as my heart hammered in my chest. I didn't have the courage to check on the SUV. *Oh my God, please let them be okay.* The weight bore down on my chest as I struggled to breathe. It was more than I could bear. Dumbfounded and feeling so much guilt within me, I staggered over to the side of my totaled car.

As hard as it was for me to call Chris and tell him that I caused an accident, I knew I had to. When I told him where I was, he was already in his car, on his way to me. After hanging up, I just stood there, trembling. I don't know how many minutes passed and I didn't know what to do but stare at my totaled car.

A short distance away, I saw Chris slowly emerge through the debris. Suddenly, I felt nauseous as my body turned into violent shakes. He looked me over carefully and pulled me close to him. I sobbed in his chest, apologizing over and over. He kept telling me that it was just an accident and everyone was okay. He helped me sit down and I took in the entire scene in front of me for the first time. There were people all over the place with two fire trucks, an ambulance, and a highway patrol car. I started gasping for air and Chris pushed my head down between my knees and helped me breathe. A paramedic came over and checked my vitals. She took care of the burn on my arm that was probably caused from the air bag. She told me how lucky I was to walk away from this head-on collision. I found out the mother and her child were fine and had already left and the young man was being taken to the E.R. to get checked over. I refused to go to the hospital. I didn't want to cause any more stress for Chris.

When we got home, I went into the bathroom and didn't recognize myself. My eyes were bloodshot, my face was streaked from the tears, my hair was in a tangled mess, and I had black specks all over my body. I threw off my clothes and stood in the shower, letting the hot water massage my head, neck, and back. I took my time, hoping I could find my escape from the reality, but it was pointless. When I opened the bathroom door, I found Chris sitting on the bed. He patted the empty space next to him and held me close.

"Steph, it was an accident. It happens sometimes and that's why we call them accidents. More than anything I'm relieved you're okay. I can replace the car, but I can't replace my girl." He kissed my forehead, the tip of my nose, and then my lips. "I don't want you to worry about anything. It's my job to take care of my wife."

"You already take care of me, Chris," I said, leaning my head on his shoulder, while he stroked my hair. I worried about him dealing with my accident during the radiation treatments. I couldn't stop thinking about the people I had hurt. I wondered if I would be able to overcome my fears about driving. I was so tired of worrying, I prayed for strength and healing from all of this.

It seemed that once the fire started, it was hard to control it. Sometimes, you just have to let it burn itself out.

Several nights later, Chris woke up feeling pressure in his bladder. We worked together to flush the catheter but it was severely blocked. By 4 a.m., I drove Chris to the E.R. Thankfully, he was taken care of right away and we found out that a blood clot had caused the blockage in the tube. *A blood clot? What does this mean?*

Early the next evening, Chris started having painful bladder spasms and the tube was blocked again. We went back to the E.R. and discovered another blood clot. *Oh God, what's happening to my husband?!* The doctor ordered a urine test and found out there was another urinary tract infection. Chris was given antibiotics and after we got home, he finally found relief and fell asleep on the couch.

When we saw Dr. Chehval the following week, he told us that the blood clot was probably from the bladder's irritation and sensitivity from the catheter. He showed Chris how to deflate the balloon and irrigate the tube and gave him extra syringes, saline solution, lubricant, tubes, and a bag.

Chris was able to continue the Hydroxyurea and Bleomycin even though the red cell counts slightly dropped and he was down another six pounds, weighing at 152 pounds. The pain medications helped reduce the pain, however Chris started having bad dreams and sudden twitches in his arms and legs. Dr. Needles adjusted the medication, hoping it would reduce those symptoms.

Chris completed the radiation by mid-November. We prayed that the tumors had been destroyed and his body would heal without any infection or more pain. We continued to explore different ways for him to sit or lie down comfortably each night, resulting in about one-to-three hours of sleep. While Chris was getting weaker, I was running out of ideas of how to help my husband, feeling more and more frustrated. But we kept riding on together through the flames, depending on God for the strength we needed and knowing He was just ahead of us to keep following Him.

"Jesus said, 'By trusting in me, you will be unshakable and assured, deeply at peace. In this world you will continue to experience difficulties. But take heart! I've conquered the world.'"

- John 16:33

A week after completing the radiation, Chris had a full morning of appointments with all three doctors. When he saw Dr. Chehval for a catheter change, he noticed the tumors had shrunk considerably and encouraged us to keep hanging in there. Chris had blood work and then saw Dr. Needles. After examining Chris, he, too, was hopeful that the tumors had shrunk. He wasn't sure if it was the radiation or the chemo or both, but it was promising. However, Chris was still in a lot of pain and Dr. Needles re-adjusted the pain medication. The blood work showed that the red cell counts dropped again, so Dr. Needles gave Chris an Aranis injection to help boost the counts and continued the next round of chemo. Dr. O'Brian thought the tumors had shrunk significantly and pointed out that a lot of new skin was already developing in the area. He suggested exposing the burns to the air while still using the ointments he had given him. Even though Chris was uncomfortable, he walked out of the cancer center tall and proud.

Mark and Toni came in town to celebrate Thanksgiving with us and my family. Everyone was surprised at how much weight Chris had lost and how tired he looked, but they offered their support and encouragement. Those positive words renewed Chris' perseverance to keep riding on.

After the holiday, we returned to Dr. O'Brian and he gave us the same report – the new skin was healthy and forming well, there were no signs of infection, and it would take time for his body to heal. We were beginning to learn a new definition of patience to get through the days and nights finding ways for Chris sit and lie down comfortably. When nothing worked, he would kneel on a cushion and rest his elbows on a pillow on the coffee table. He talked on the phone, watched television, read, ate and even slept kneeling. Whenever his knees would get tired, I'd stack all of our cushions and pillows on the couch along the wall and he'd lean against them and sleep without ever falling down. I'd camp out with him and wake up often through the night to check on him. Sometimes, he slept about two hours and other nights, it would be three to four hours. Chris told me how he used to take naps during his tours of duty in the Navy when he worked long hours. Whenever he had a break, he'd go to a place where it was quiet, fold his arms across his chest, and lean against the wall with his feet slightly apart to maintain balance and take a brief nap. He would actually sleep and when he woke up, he felt rested enough to go back to work.

By the beginning of December, fatigue was catching up to the both of us. Chris was getting weaker and I barely kept up with my lesson plans, assessments, paper work, and meetings. I was so worried about Chris that I wanted to go with him to see Dr. Needles, however he insisted that I save my day for when we needed it most.

After dismissal, I checked my voicemail and found out Chris was going to be admitted to the hospital. Feeling the panic rise inside my chest, my fingers shook as I dialed Chris' number.

"Chris, what's wrong?"

"Hi Steph, I'm at the cancer center. My red cell count is really low and I'm anemic so I have to have a blood transfusion."

"Are you okay? Are you in a lot of pain? Are you..."

"Steph, I'm fine." Chris interrupted. "I'll wait for you here and we'll go over to the hospital together. Take your time. I want you to drive safely."

I grabbed my things and rushed down the stairs to my car. I fought back the tears and gripped the steering wheel to steady my fingers. I chided myself for not following my instincts to go to the appointment with Chris. The rush-hour traffic was moving along smoothly and I was able to get there in no time. I parked in front of the main entrance of the cancer center and ran into the building and up three flights of stairs. I hurried through the doors into the chemo treatment room and stopped breathlessly in front of Chris, sleeping in a recliner. *Oh God. He looks so fragile and worn out.* Chris opened one of his eyes and smiled.

"Hi sweetie," he said.

"You are too cute," I whispered. A nurse came over with a glass of water for me and patted my shoulder.

"Chris is okay, Stephanie," she said calmly. "His red cell count is low and he has a mild fever. Dr. Needles wants to admit Chris to the hospital and run some tests to find out what's causing the temperature and to get a blood transfusion."

"I didn't want to go to the E.R. without you," Chris said. "I knew you'd be worried and I didn't want you to drive here in that state of mind." I shook my head thinking how he was so concerned about me when he should've gone to the hospital already.

"Okay, Chris. So how about we get over to the E.R."

The staff admitted him right away, started the fluids and began some tests. While I was waiting for Chris to return, his cell phone rang and it was Pat, already at our house. I had forgotten he was flying in from Washington State to spend a few days with us. I explained what was going on and he told me he would meet us at the hospital. By the time Pat arrived, Chris was already settled in his room.

"Hey man," Chris smiled and they shook hands.

"You get yourself admitted to the hospital when you knew I was coming in town, Chris? What's up with that?" Pat joked. They hadn't seen each other since our wedding day. It was great watching them catch up and the special bond they shared.

Over the next couple of days, Chris had to have three units of blood while Pat stayed and kept him company. We found out there was a mild staph infection in the urinary tract. *Oh God, this is beyond what Chris and I can handle. But You can take care of this.*

Since we caught it early, Chris wouldn't have to repeat the same antibiotic treatment as the year before. He was prescribed to take a pill daily for two weeks. *Thank you, Lord!*

After two days in the hospital, Chris' blood count was normal and he was released to go home. Unfortunately, it was time for Pat to go back home too. Chris felt bad that they had to spend time together in the hospital, but Pat helped renew his strength to keep on fighting.

A week later, Chris was feeling better again. He started getting into the spirit of the season and wanted to decorate our Christmas tree, feeling the miracle of Christmas and the hope of beating the cancer. I worried he might overdo it, but I couldn't say no to him.

One morning, Chris went to a get-together at the Missouri State Highway Patrol and reunited with many of the men he used to work with. When I got home, he was sitting on the couch, very quiet and solemn. My hands balled up into fists, ready to deal with what could be wrong. I sat next to my husband and waited until he was ready.

"Steph, when I went to the Christmas party this morning, everyone was happy to see me. They were so kind and went out of their way to make sure I was comfortable." He wiped his eyes. "They really cared, Steph." I don't know if Chris had ever felt this kind of compassion from his colleagues before. I realized he needed this act of tender loving care from his patrol and I thanked God for bringing him to that party.

"Goodness and mercy shall follow me all the days of my life."

- Psalm 23:6

A week before Christmas, we met with Dr. Needles to find out the results of the MRI. We couldn't wait to hear the good news, feeling hopeful that we finally had control over the cancer.

"Well," Dr. Needles paused, "it looks like there is significant shrinkage of the tumors. However there is a lot of haziness due to the inflammation in the area from the radiation, but from what we can tell the tumor in the perineum shrunk about 4 centimeters and another has shrunk about 3 centimeters." *Oh, thank you God!*

Dr. Needles wasn't sure if it was the radiation, the chemo, or both so it was hard to determine which method of treatment worked. Chris started back on the Hydroxyurea and Dr. Needles wanted to do a pulmonary function test to check Chris' lung capacity before starting

Bleomycin again. We were rescheduled to return after the New Year to find out.

After seeing Dr. Needles, Chris had a follow-up appointment with Dr. O'Brian. It had been almost three weeks since he last saw him. He assured us that Chris was healing well and more new skin was growing. I tried to get him to understand how hard it had been for Chris to sit, lie down, and walk comfortably and that he hadn't been able to get any rest. He encouraged us to be patient for his body to recover. I helped Chris back to the car, feeling more frustrated, alone, and most of all helpless. It's the worse feeling when you don't know what you can do to relieve your loved one's pain. Fighting back the tears, I prayed as I drove us home.

We can be patient, but God, how do we get through this?

Storms

"Haven't I commanded you? Strength. Courage. Do not be afraid. Don't get discouraged. Your God is with you every step you take."
- Joshua 1:9

Over the holidays, the pulmonary function test showed nothing wrong with Chris' lung function or capacity and Chris gained his weight back to 170 pounds. His red cell count dropped slightly and he had another Aranis shot to try to boost it back up. Dr. Needles resumed Hydroxyurea daily and Bleomycin once every two weeks. Dr. O'Brian showed Chris where more healthy skin was growing and suggested a different way to treat the wounds. However, the pain became so unbearable, Chris went back to the way he had been treating the burns before.

The dreary days in January seemed to reflect our struggle to keep on pedaling. Chris was in constant pain with very little rest and when he did sleep, it was preoccupied with vivid dreams.

The first time, Chris dreamt that D'Artagnon had been severely hurt and was dying. He woke up crying out for his dog and I couldn't console him. Worried that something was really wrong with D'Artagnon, I checked on him and he was curled up like a big ball of fur, sleeping soundly. Chris finally calmed down and eventually fell back asleep.

Another time, Chris woke me up kicking and punching wildly in the air. I had a hard time waking him up out of his dream. He searched around the bedroom with wide and fearful eyes.

"Are you okay?" he asked, checking me over.

"I'm fine Chris." He broke into tears and held me for a long time.

"I was fighting a burglar in our house, protecting you. Steph, it was so real."

"Oh babe, it was just a dream. We're all safe. Only a fool would try to break into this house with D'Artagnon and two yappy little dogs." We started laughing and calmed down. Chris fell back asleep while I stayed awake, stroking his eyebrows and praying for God's supernatural protection over Chris.

Fortunately he didn't remember either of those dreams.

One day, Chris dozed off while he was changing the bandages and fell through the shower doors in our bathroom. He knocked them out of the groove, but luckily the glass didn't break and Chris wasn't hurt. I begged him to let me help, but he refused to let me see the burns.

I went with Chris to his appointments with the three doctors, determined to find relief for him. We discovered he had another urinary tract infection and Dr. Chehval prescribed antibiotics. Dr. Needles re-adjusted the pain medication and we learned that Chris' red cell count had dropped again and he had to get another blood transfusion. Chris' legs and feet were swollen, making him feel stiff and harder to move around. Dr. O'Brian suggested taking a break from the chemo and ordered a test to check for blood clots.

Even though we rode through many obstacles in this race, this particular course was the most challenging. It felt like we were riding through a long, drawn-out storm, dealing with so much pain and restless nights. I knew Chris rode in the rain many times, but did he know how to endure a storm?

One day, Father Don, our parish priest, talked about how to get through the storms that occur in our lives. We had just heard the story when Jesus and his disciples were stuck in the middle of a terrible storm – something akin to a hurricane. The boat thrashed back and forth, filling up with water, and the disciples were losing control. They looked for Jesus to help them and he was sleeping. How could he be sleeping?! Didn't he know they were in the middle of a great storm? Didn't he care about the danger they were in?

- Matthew 8:23 – 27; Mark 4:35 – 41; or Luke 8:22 – 25

"Does this sound familiar to you?" Father Don inquired. "Perhaps you've asked the same questions: 'Where is Jesus in all of this? Why is He so silent that we cannot hear Him? Doesn't He care that we're afraid or suffering?'" he paused before continuing on.

"We tend to forget that Jesus is always there in the middle of our storms. He would never abandon us.

The question to ask Him shouldn't be: 'Where are you, Jesus, in all of this?'

The questions we should ask are: 'Where am I in the middle of this storm? Am I willing to trust God through this storm? Am I willing to reach out to others? Am I willing to put myself in the middle of another's storm – exposing my own vulnerability – not knowing what to say or do, but rather be there for another – to offer my love, hope, comfort, encouragement, help, and support?'

We are vulnerable to the storms in our lives, however if we remember that God is right here with us and trust in Him, our vulnerability turns into grace and God gives us strength to endure and persevere through the storm.

Jesus asks us to answer two questions: Who is responsible for all of the world and creation? In whose hands are you right now? Jesus believes that our answer to these two questions have the power not to take away the storm, but to quiet the panic within us. The storms will always come and go. What remains constant is that we remain in God's hands."

I truly believe God sent certain people at the right moment to help calm the storm around us and renew our strength.

"Anyone who is having troubles, should pray. He cares for you."

- James 5:13 and 1ˢᵗ Peter 5:7

Toward the end of January, Bob, Kelly, and their kids spent an afternoon with us, sharing their encouragement, energy, optimism, and sense of humor. Their visit re-energized us to keep going.

Several days later, Mark and Toni spent a few days with us. At first, it was hard when they saw how difficult our fight had become. They noticed how fatigued and weak Chris was, the amount of time he spent in the bathroom taking care of his wounds, and how difficult it was for him to move, sit, and lay down. They helped Chris as much as they could and gave me new ideas and questions for the doctors.

After these visits, I realized Chris needed more prayers and support to keep riding on in his race. I sent out another e-mail to our friends and families with suggestions on how to be there for Chris.

It was amazing to see the hand of God at work. Our neighbors took turns to have lunch with Chris. Mark and Toni suggested massage treatments for Chris' legs which led Dr. Needles to wonder if the swelling is caused from stress or scar tissue from the radiation – and ordered physical therapy for him. Dr. Needles and Dr. Chehval worked together to figure out a different pain regimen to help Chris relieve his pain and get better sleep at night. I asked about getting home health care assistance since Chris refused to let me help him. Dr. O'Brian agreed and put in an order for a wound care specialist. Through all of these changes, I prayed thanks to God for hearing us and continued believing for complete healing from the cancer.

We found out there were no blood clots and the insurance company approved physical therapy and home care. A week later, a wound care nurse who specialized in burn care evaluated Chris and scheduled to see him twice a week.

After her second visit, Chris learned new ways of bandaging with different ointments and materials that made it less painful for him. She suggested Chris try a firm mattress to sleep on. I removed the mattress from the bed in the guest bedroom and put the futon mattress on it. When Chris laid down, he slept for five-and-a-half hours without waking up – the first time in a long, long time.

With the heaviest storms in January behind us, I looked forward to the clouds breaking up as things started improving for Chris. I gave God praise for His goodness and mercy on my husband.

Chris started physical therapy on Presidents' Day and I was able to go with him to meet his therapist. She went through a round of questions and evaluated his legs. She recommended leg massages twice a week to reduce the swelling and improve the circulation in them. She warned us that it would be a long time before Chris would be ready for actual physical therapy.

Within a couple of weeks, Chris' schedule became full with the wound care nurse, the physical therapist, Dr. Needles, Dr. Chehval, and our neighbors' visits. I was thrilled he was around positive and supportive people to help him keep riding on in his race. Chris started receiving get well cards from our families, friends, co-workers, and people we didn't know who were thinking of him. He was deeply touched when they shared their hope, encouragement, and prayers for him. He especially loved the jokes in some of the cards.

By mid-February, we met with Dr. Needles to hear the results from the MRI and CT-scan.

"How have you been feeling, Chris?" Dr. Needles asked and Chris filled him in.

"Good, I'm glad everything is starting to get better for you," Dr. Needles smiled and opened Chris' growing file.

"The MRI was hazy due to the inflammation from the radiation burns. However it appears that there are dead tissues where the tumors once were." *Oh God, thank you!*

"But…"

What? No. No "buts."

"...the CT-scan of your chest," Dr. Needles paused, looking at Chris, "showed more tumor activity from the nodules and one of them measures about a centimeter."

How does one handle feeling leaps of joy to bearing a heavy weight in your heart in a matter of seconds?

Since Chris was scheduled for another cystoscopy to check his bladder and remove some scar tissue, Dr. Needles wanted to consult with Dr. Chehval and some of the other doctors before deciding what to do next.

"It's going to be okay, Steph," Chris said optimistically.

I trust you, God. You know what to do. All things are possible with You especially when they seem impossible to us.

Walking out of the cancer center into the sunshine, I felt a sense of peace within my heart. It was as if God answered me: *No worries my child, I will get you through this.*

Two days later, we were back at the surgery center for the cystoscopy. After Chris was settled on the gurney, Dr. Chehval came by to check on him and jotted some notes in his chart. Before I knew it, the anesthesiologist – one we didn't know – gave Chris the "happy" medicine without giving us a chance to kiss each other goodbye. I stood in the middle of the hall and watched my husband disappear in the surgery room. I took a deep breath and walked slowly back to the waiting room to sit with Poppa Bob who was free to keep me company. I knew in my heart Chris was in God's hands and I prayed for Him to work through Dr. Chehval to take care of him. We didn't wait long when Dr. Chehval came out and sat next to me.

"Chris is doing fine. I didn't see any signs of cancer," he smiled, patting my hand. "I was able to remove some scar tissue around the perineum which should make things easier for Chris." I thanked Dr. Chehval and hugged him.

"Well, I'd say it's about time you two had some really good news," Poppa said.

Several days later, the wound care nurse noticed the wounds in the perineum were healing much better and Chris told her it had been easier to move around again. I was thrilled to see things getting better for him.

When we returned to Dr. Needles, he was pleased with the cystoscopy report, but he was still concerned about the spots in Chris' lungs. After reviewing everything, he suggested staying on

Hydroxyurea and Bleomycin treatments since Chris had been off of it for over a month to give his body time to heal from the burns. Dr. Needles wanted to do the chemo for about two months and then go from there. Chris was all for it. There was a new sense of energy in him as if he was back on the bike and pedaling strong to keep going in his race.

Throughout March, Chris adapted to his routine with the visits from the wound care nurse and our neighbors, going to physical therapy twice a week, checking his blood counts once a week, and seeing Dr. Chehval every two weeks to change the catheter. He rode on with it, doing whatever he had to do to get better and fight the cancer. Since Chris was constantly around people, it became easier for me to focus on my job at the end of the third quarter: grading assessments, completing report cards, and meeting with parents for conferences.

By the end of the month, Chris started experiencing sudden jerks in his hands and legs and sometimes his pulse would race to the point that it made him breathless. The physical dreams were back causing Chris to have restless nights again. Dr. Needles felt that the pain medicine was causing these symptoms and re-adjusted the dosage. As the twitches and dreams subsided, Chris began having painful bladder spasms again. He called Dr. Chehval who prescribed antibiotics right away, thinking it was another urinary tract infection. Usually Chris would find relief within 24 hours, but the spasms continued with a vengeance.

It seemed like we would resolve one problem and then another problem would flare up. It felt like we couldn't catch a break, going through one storm to the next. I went with Chris for his appointments during the first week of April to find out what we could do for him. Dr. Chehval ordered another urine culture and wrote a different prescription for the spasms, hoping it would help Chris.

Chris told Dr. Needles that the pain medicine was working better since he didn't have the sudden jerks or active dreams anymore. Chris' red cell count was stable and he was able to continue the chemo. Dr. Needles ordered a CT-scan and another pulmonary function test to re-assess his lungs.

During the meeting with Chris' physical therapist, we found out he was ready to do exercises. Chris was overly enthusiastic and attempted to do an extra set of everything she had him do, but she advised him to take it slow on the first day and promised to add an extra set for the next visit.

It had been such a long stretch and the storms had finally passed over. I knew we still had a long way to go, but I felt more hopeful that things would continue to get better for Chris.

Enduring the Trials

If you have fallen and feel like you have reached the lowest point in your race, stretch out your hands and God will pull you up. Brush yourself off and keep going as best as you can. God will take care of the rest.

Chris continued to struggle through the following days and nights while the radiation burns were healing. He was still having a lot of pain from the creases and dealing with sudden bladder spasms. Fortunately, there were no signs of an infection. Chris kept up with his physical therapy exercises at home and I'd help him stretch before and after school and before going to bed. Soon he was able to drive, regaining a sense of independence.

Everyday, when I came home, Chris would tell me, "Today is a good day, Steph." He didn't let anything keep him from living each day as best as he could. On the better days, it was as if he was coasting on the road, feeling the freedom of the wind. When he was having a hard day, he would grip the handlebars and press forward, riding on without giving up.

By mid-April, I went with Chris again for his physical therapy session and to meet with Dr. Needles. I watched him work out and was amazed at how far he had come after five visits. No matter what he had to do, Chris rose to each challenge above and beyond. When his therapist told him to do something 12 times, he'd do 15. When he was out of earshot, she told me he was one of her favorite clients – always cooperative, followed through on his daily stretches and exercises at home, stayed optimistic and positive, and worked hard to get better.

"Chris, I would like to get you on a stationery bike and some other exercise machines." He suddenly stopped and his face lit up like a little boy. The joy and excitement he showed brought me to tears, I had to look away to compose myself. It had been almost two years since Chris had been on a bike. I couldn't imagine him going through another summer without riding again. This would be a great first step in getting him back on his bike.

"Okay," she laughed, "I would need you to get Dr. Needles to write up the order for physical therapy at the rehab gym."

"No problem," Chris said confidently and resumed his exercise. Even though he was worn out, he was practically bouncing in his walk when we went to get blood work done at Dr. Needles' office. He couldn't stop smiling. *Oh God, thank you for hearing our prayers.*

While we waited for Dr. Needles, Chris sat comfortably in the chair, relaxed with his eyes closed. It was such a relief to see him sit again without any problems. Chris opened his eyes and looked at me with a silly grin.

"What's up?" he asked.

"Nothing. I'm just looking at my triple H hubby."

"Huh?" I laughed at his confused expression and explained what I meant.

"I'm looking at my healthy, handsome, hunk of a husband."

"Funny girl," he said, shaking his head. The door opened suddenly and Dr. Needles walked quickly into the room.

"How have you been doing, Chris?" he asked. Chris told him about the bladder spasms and dealing with pain from the creases. Dr. Needles modified the pain medicine again. He was pleased to hear how physical therapy was going and agreed to write an order for therapy at the rehab gym. He paused and opened the dreaded file. I couldn't help but sense that something wasn't right. I gripped my pen and waited for Dr. Needles to break the deafening silence in the small room.

"The CT-scan showed many more nodules in both lungs. Most are less than three centimeters and some are a little larger. It's obvious that the Hydroxyurea and Bleomycin are not working."

We sat there, speechless. I felt another heavy weight of this cancer bearing down on me, making it almost too much to handle. *How dare this cancer consume my husband's body?* I wanted it to leave Chris alone.

After several minutes, Chris cleared his throat.

"Doctor, what can I do now?" he asked. Dr. Needles suggested trying Gemzar (which was what we used in the first treatment) with Carboplatin – a new chemo we hadn't tried yet. But we had to wait for the insurance to approve it and Dr. Needles wanted Chris to have a week off to recuperate from the Hydroxyurea.

"Steph, it's going to be okay." Chris said. I nodded, not trusting myself to speak.

When we got home, Chris went to the bathroom to change his bandages and I stayed outside with the dogs, hoping the air would clear my mind. I realized I let my anger overwhelm me, which made me forget Chris' feelings. I lifted my arms like wings toward the bright, blue sky, leaned my head back to feel the sun's warmth on my face, took in a slow deep breath and then exhaled. *God, help me to understand and know how to give up my worries, fear, and anger to You right away. I don't want to be stuck in the dark. Let Your Light shine on me. Help me with the kind of wisdom to see things Your way – no matter what happens – and fight the good fight of my faith in You.*

I knew I had fallen off my bike. So, I picked myself up, hiked back up on the seat and started pedaling to catch up to my husband.

I went inside to find Chris.

"Come sit next to me," he said, patting the empty spot on the couch. "Steph, you know how much I love you. I'm so lucky to have a woman like you who loves me just as much. I know you're doing everything you can to take care of me. You have become more than I ever hoped for and prayed for as my best friend and as my wife. I wouldn't have been able to keep going in this fight without you by my side. I know the news today really upset you and you're trying to be strong for me. I want to thank you for that. But I can't handle it if you keep your thoughts and feelings from me. Steph, we're in this together, from the start to the finish. We will get through it. It's going to be okay. I don't know how I know it, I just do, Steph. This cancer will not destroy my will to fight, to live, to hope, or to love you each day."

The love I felt from Chris and had for him was the kind of love that gave us strength and courage, peace and contentment, and true happiness. It grew deeply between us because we felt God's love within our love for one another and it was an incredible joy that superseded our hopes and dreams.

"We have not seen God and yet we love Him; even without seeing Him, we believe in Him and experience a heavenly joy beyond all words, for we are reaching the goal of our faith: the salvation of our souls."

- 1st Peter 1:8 – 9

I told Chris how I felt since hearing the news and to my surprise, he admitted to getting angry at the cancer sometimes.

"But I just let it go, because I know God can handle it much better than me. He knows what to do about it," Chris said.

"Cast your burden on the Lord, and He shall sustain you; He shall never permit the righteous to be moved. [He will not let you fail]."
- Psalm 55:22

We kept riding on, taking it one day at a time. The week flew by and Chris had another busy day with three appointments. He wanted me to work in the morning and meet him at Dr. Needles' office in the afternoon. When I got there, he was in the waiting room and told me about his morning.

"Dr. Chehval changed the tube and ordered another urine culture to see if I have an infection. He gave me new samples to try for the spasms. But my physical therapy was great, Steph. I get to start at the rehab gym next week," he said excitedly.

Chris' weight was stable and his blood counts were good. The insurance company approved the chemo and Chris would get Gemzar and Carboplatin once a week for two weeks, take a week break, and repeat the course three more times. We scheduled the next seven appointments from May through June, feeling especially hopeful this regimen was going to work. It had been over two years since we had started on this journey. This time, he just *had* to get better.

After the first round, Chris didn't have much of an appetite and he took more naps. He kept on going as best as he could with his routine, always looking forward to being healed from the cancer.

Several days later, Mark and Toni stopped by for a short visit. Even though Chris was still tired from the chemo treatment, he enjoyed every minute, laughing and sharing stories with his family.

By the weekend, Chris gained some of his strength back and woke up feeling better than he had felt in a long time. We celebrated Mother's Day and my birthday with Bob's family and my family. Chris didn't have any pain or discomfort. It was the best birthday present I could ever hope for and kept thanking God for giving Chris an exceptional day. He even stood in front of everyone and sang his special birthday song to me. I turned my wish into a prayer for a complete healing and recovery from the cancer before blowing out the candles. Watching the smoke billow up and disappear, I imagined my prayer went straight up to God, with hope in my heart.

The next morning, Chris woke up with painful bladder spasms again and discovered a blood clot in the tube when he flushed it out. He called Dr. Chehval who prescribed antibiotics and a new medicine for the spasms. A couple of days later, the spasms went away, just in time when Michael came to visit us.

One evening, we were talking about our faith.

"Chris, your strength and positive attitude inspires so many of us in the way you keep going in your fight. Steph, your love for my brother and how you stand by his side through everything shows us how we should take care of each other. Chris, Steph, you have a very special story," Michael said.

We didn't know what to say. We had been so consumed in our fight against the cancer, we didn't realize how others saw us in our race or how we affected them. Later that night, Chris and I explored the idea of writing a book. We remembered when Fitz and Teddie Momma told us that we were witnesses for each other and had a testimony about our faith, hope, and love for others. *Would anyone be interested in a story about us?* We agreed that it was something to really think about and talk over later on, after we beat this cancer.

Several days later, Michael left to get back to work. Chris was very quiet, watching his younger brother drive off, and wiped his eyes. The past two weeks were some of the happiest in his life, I prayed for more of these days for him.

We spent the rest of the weekend going out to eat and taking short walks, enjoying the warm, spring weather. Then it was back to reality for the second round of chemo. Even though it made him tired, Chris kept up his exercises as I helped him stretch every day. The wound care nurse continued to check on Chris twice a week since he was still having pain from the creases which were the hardest areas to heal. She encouraged Chris to remain patient through the healing process.

Chris decided he wanted to join a cancer support group at a local church. He loved hearing God's Word and felt more inspired to fight the good fight of his faith in Him. People gravitated to Chris after hearing how much he had been through and how strong his faith was in God. He didn't realize how much he helped them to keep going in their own race since they had given him the kind of encouragement he needed to stay strong.

As Chris continued feeling better, he started taking me out on dates again. We went to the movies, picnics in the park, and to Fritz's.

Bob and Kelly hosted their annual 5K walk/run fundraiser at their gym and chose to sponsor Chris again. Some of Chris' family came to participate in the event along with many of our friends, gym members, and competitive runners. Chris was overwhelmed by the words of encouragement, support, and prayers from everyone.

Later, I found Chris standing by himself off to the side, watching the participants get ready at the starting line. My heart ached as I remembered when Chris told me he would run this year to help someone else in their fight. I squeezed his hand and he looked at me.

"Next year, Chris," I said confidently. He smiled and squeezed my hand back.

Several days later, Chris took me out to a special dinner for our second wedding anniversary. He was just as excited as I was and dressed up as well as he could in loose-fitting khaki pants with a deep red polo shirt. It didn't matter what he wore, my husband could look good in anything. He took me to a local golf club restaurant that overlooked a lake. As the sun dropped in the horizon during our meal, the reflection of the orange and purple skies in the water was mesmerizing, creating a soft glow on our faces.

"To my wife who has become my angel on earth," Chris said, raising his glass to me. "Happy Second Anniversary." I wrapped my glass around his and kissed him.

"I treasure every moment we share together. I love you more today than yesterday and I can't wait to love you again tomorrow."

God blessed us with more exceptional days throughout June as Chris got stronger and better. It had been a very long and rough road since the radiation treatment in November and it felt like we were riding in the light of hope.

Chris continued to improve in his physical therapy at the rehab gym. When I got home, he told me about his first work out.

"Steph, it felt like home sitting on the exercise bike. I rode two miles on it today," he told me proudly.

"Soon, you'll be able to ride your own bike Chris," I said and his eyes lit up. We gave God praise for being so good to us.

Chris completed the last round of Gemzar and Carboplatin and Dr. Needles ordered another MRI and CT-scan. Chris' white cell count had dropped significantly which indicated another urinary tract infection and he was put on antibiotics again. I wondered if he would have to stay on it as long as he had the suprapubic catheter. I prayed for God to heal this infection permanently and truly believed He had already taken care of it. We had to wait a couple of weeks before we would know the results of the tests. We forgot what it was like to go through a long waiting period and made the best of each day. In the meantime, Chris started coughing and he insisted it was just a summer cold, nothing serious especially since his white cell count was low. After a week, the coughing subsided and I thought maybe Chris was right.

We started talking about our future, excited to look beyond our victory over the cancer – we were that confident Chris would be healed. It felt right to think about starting our family, even though we were still riding on in this race. The thought of having a baby made us giggle with so much joy, we couldn't wait. We decided to pray more about it to make sure it was the right thing for us to do.

"I watch in hope for the Lord, I wait for God my Savior. My God will hear me."

- Micah 7:7

"As Long as You Keep Fighting..."

"When the world says, 'Give up,' Hope whispers, 'Try it one more time.'"

- Author Unknown

Chris was making more progress from physical therapy and was able to move around easily, even with the suprapubic catheter. One day I heard him call me from the bedroom and when I rushed in, he was smiling.

"Watch this, Steph," he said excitedly. He bent down, touched his feet, put on his tennis shoes and tied the laces by himself. I'd been helping him with his shoes since October. We thanked God for this great feat and decided to celebrate by going on a picnic lunch and to Fritz's ice cream for dessert.

During the second week of July, we were back at Dr. Needles' office again. He was pleased at how well Chris had been doing and then told us the results of the tests.

"The MRI showed some kind of activity in the penis and scrotum."

What does that mean? Another tumor? Oh God.

Neither of us said anything and I struggled to stay strong for the both of us.

"But there is some fluid in the scrotum which could be inflammation from the radiation. We'll keep an eye on it." Dr. Needles paused, looking over his notes. "The CT-scan showed several nodules in the lungs grew, with the largest measuring at four centimeters and the smallest at two centimeters. I suggest trying a different regimen using Camptosar with 5-Fluorourocil," he said and focused on Chris. "You would start the treatment here and continue it with a chemo pump for another 46 hours at home. You will have a two-week break in between each round. I would like to try four courses of it."

"When can I start?" Chris asked, breaking the eerie silence in the room.

"Today," Dr. Needles answered, handing the order to me. Before walking out the door, he turned around. "Chris," he paused and we looked up at him, "as long as you keep fighting, I will keep fighting for you." With wide eyes and my mouth agape, I slowly turned to my husband. He slapped his knees and stood up quickly.

"Let's do it," he said optimistically. Smiling, both men nodded. Chris glanced down at me and put his hands on his hips.

"Well, are you ready?" he asked. Still in a state of awe, I quickly packed our things in the backpack.

"I knew I chose the right doctor," he said.

Yes you did, Chris! I wondered if any other doctor would have given up by now. Shivering at the thought, I disregarded it and thanked God for Dr. Needles. While Chris decided which recliner to use, I handed the order to a nurse who pulled me aside where he couldn't hear her.

"Stephanie, I was really worried about Chris several months ago and I'm so happy to see him doing well. He has such a great positive and optimistic attitude. It's part of the fight to stay hopeful. I believe Chris will beat it." I looked over at my husband, anxious to get started.

"Chris is already beating it," I said, smiling at her.

We joined Chris and she explained how the chemo pump worked while connecting the I.V. from the port in his chest to the pump, but it didn't faze him.

"Hey, if I could put up with a picc line for two months, this will be a piece of cake to deal with for two days," he said. "Hey, speaking of cake, Steph do you think you could make those chocolate cupcakes I love so much?" We started laughing and Chris promised to bring his nurse one when he came back. I found out that the most common side effects of these two chemo drugs were fatigue and loss of appetite. I would have to bake those cupcakes as soon as we got home.

Over the next two hours, Chris slept while I prayed fervently.

God, thank you for a doctor who cares so much for Chris that he continues fighting for him. Let this chemo be the right one to destroy the cancer. I know you can heal Chris' body from the cancer and all of the chemo and radiation he had been through. You said, "For humans it is impossible, but for You, Oh God, all things are possible." As long as we keep on fighting and believing in our faith, hope, and love, I know You will keep on fighting for us. Having You within our spirit is so much greater and more powerful than the cancer.

I asked God again for guidance and strength to keep riding on in this leg of our race. I prayed for an abundance of His love through it all so that Chris and I could share our love for each other and for Him. I thanked God for giving us the power, love, and a sound mind that was beyond our understanding as we continue to put our faith and hope in Him.

Before leaving the cancer center, the nurse put the pump in a small bag with a long handle so Chris could easily carry it over his shoulder.

"It's like you have your own man purse," I teased. Chris pretended to look in the bag for something and acted like he found it. He puckered his lips and demonstrated putting on lipstick. He leaned over and kissed me quickly.

"You are such a clown," I laughed. But he wasn't finished. He looked in the bag again and pretended to file his nails, blinking his eyelashes.

After 24-hours of the chemo, fatigue overwhelmed Chris and he slept most of the second day. I drove him back to the cancer center to have the pump removed and a couple of days later he bounced back to his old self. However, Chris started having some swelling in the scrotum. When he saw Dr. Chehval to replace the catheter tube, he thought it might be fluid, but didn't want to drain it while on chemo. He offered suggestions to help Chris relieve some of the discomfort.

As we continued to take each day at a time, we talked and prayed more about having a family. We strongly felt that it was the right time and met with our fertility doctor at the end of July. She suggested trying In-Vitro Fertilization. I couldn't believe how much I had to do to prepare my body for the procedure: the constant blood work (*I hate needles*) and ultrasounds, the medicine I would have to take and the injections I'd have to give myself (*oh boy*), and the surgical procedures to remove my eggs and implant the embryos. Then she told us that there was a strong possibility we could have twins.

Twins? I looked at Chris who was beaming. *Oh God, what a wonderful gift I could give to my husband.* We were so excited to have two babies that it felt like we were floating on a cloud. We imagined the possibility of having a boy and a girl and started brainstorming names for them. Chris was so happy, you would have thought he was already a daddy. The last time he was this ecstatic was on our wedding day.

Several days later, I had an ultrasound and did a trial embryo transfer procedure. The technician and the doctor were pleased.

"Everything looks perfect. The embryo transfer should be simple," the doctor told us.

"Stephanie, you have a beautiful uterus," the technician said. Shocked, I glanced over at Chris, who was nodding and smiling broadly.

"Could you print out the picture?" Chris asked her. She stopped and looked at him strangely. "So my wife could put it in our baby scrapbook and label it 'Vacancy – Babies Wanted Here,'" he explained. We all burst out laughing.

The next step for us was to attend an orientation meeting before starting the process. I set up all of the appointments in August: the meeting, blood work, and ultrasounds.

Things continued going well for us and we were enjoying life as much as we could. When Chris went in for the second round of chemo, his blood cell count was stable, which was unusual, so Dr. Needles decided to increase the dose of the chemo. He examined Chris and felt that the swelling in the scrotum could be from the radiation. He couldn't drain it during chemo, but gave some ideas to help reduce the swelling and discomfort.

Chris napped again during the two-hour treatment while I prayed again for complete healing and recovery from the cancer. By the evening, fatigue hit Chris hard and he slept through the night. The next day, he developed a sore in his mouth and was given a prescription. Two days later, he bounced back and the sore was healed.

Summer was winding down and it was time to set up my classroom for the new school year while Chris worked diligently to finish his models for the annual IPMS convention held at Virginia Beach. His wound care nurse came to do a final evaluation before releasing him. After six months with her, Chris was sad to see her go. She became his saving grace who helped him heal from the burns and enjoy life again.

Since it was the first contractual week of the new school year, I couldn't go with Chris to the convention, so he planned a guys' road trip. He deserved a break from the doctors and the cancer center. I prayed for a safe trip and the best time he could have with his friends.

While he was gone, we talked every morning and night and I heard in Chris' voice that he was having a great time. I thanked God he was enjoying himself. He spent a lot of time checking out the vendors and studying the different models that were entered in the contest. His hotel room overlooked the Navy Pier and he loved waking up in the morning to open the curtains and see the sun rise over the silver water, lined with ships, bringing him back to his Navy days.

I continued to believe that this chemo regimen was working in Chris' favor. I knew God's hand was all over it and He would be victorious. I felt a sense of peace within me and knew God was working for us and through us. As long as we kept pedaling on in our race, God would lead us to the finish line.

"I will guide you in the way of wisdom and lead you along straight paths. When you walk, your steps will not be hampered; when you run, you will not stumble."

- Proverbs 4:11 – 12

The third round of chemo was scheduled on my first day of school and I couldn't be with Chris. He promised that it would be okay since we knew what to expect. During the visit, Chris told Dr. Needles about the sinus problems and shortness of breath while in Virginia. Dr. Needles prescribed antibiotics for a possible sinus infection and an inhaler, but he didn't like hearing this and ordered another CT-scan of Chris' chest.

We didn't have much time to think what the CT-scan meant as my dog, Benji's health rapidly declined within a couple of days. He stopped eating, even the baby carrots he loved so much. The vet did blood work to find out what was wrong. I couldn't imagine another problem along with diabetes, cataracts, and congestive heart failure. But he was a tough little dog who kept on going and loving us every day. This little white fur ball with big brown eyes would always sit at Chris' feet to keep him company and watched over him. When I had my breakdowns, he would cuddle next to me and lick my cheek to kiss my tears away.

"I love this dog so much, Chris. I don't know what I can do to make him better," I sobbed.

"Just keep loving him, Steph." Chris said.

By the end of the week, Benji's vet called with the dreaded news. I gave the phone to Chris, while I lovingly cradled my dog. Even when I picked him up, as gently as I could, he yelped in pain. I knew he was suffering and it was time to let him go. Chris hugged Benji and me, with tears streaming down his cheeks.

"You've been such a good dog, Benji. Thank you for staying by my side all those times when I was hurting. I love you little guy."

I held him close as Chris drove us to the vet. Benji snuggled against my chest and licked my cheek. He was such a happy dog who really enjoyed his life and knew he was loved so much. The vet assured me that I had done everything I could to take good care of him and he lived longer because of my attention to him.

"I love you, Benji. Thank you for being the best dog I've ever had," I whispered, holding Benji in my arms as he took his last breath.

The hardest thing I had to do was leave my dog behind as Chris walked me out of the building. He took care of me the rest of the day while I grieved for my beloved pet. We talked about how Benji never gave up on a tug-of-war, how he ferociously shook his rope, tossed it high up in the air and caught it, and how he took his time exploring outside while ignoring us to come home until he was good and ready, staying true to his title Mark had given him, "Sir Benjamin of the Court."

When we got home, Bridget frantically searched for Benji, whining and wondering where he was until she wore herself out. Whenever we returned from the vet, she would make sure he was okay and stayed as close as she could next to him whenever he wasn't feeling well. Even though Bridget was a few years younger, she acted like she was his mother. Over the next several days, Chris and I spent a lot of time with her and D'Artagnon to help each other through our grief.

Although we were so sad, we were anxious to hear the result of the CT-scan. We focused on our hope that this chemo regimen was working against the cancer.

When Dr. Needles opened the door, he slowly walked in with his eyebrows scrunched together, creating deep creases in his forehead. Chris and I watched him carefully. With a deep sigh, he told us that the cancer had progressed since the last CT-scan at the beginning of July.

"The tumors are spreading through the lungs quickly. Several of the previous noted tumors have grown – the largest grew from four centimeters to five. And now there is some fluid in the lower right lung, which may have caused the shortness of breath you experienced in Virginia." Dr. Needles paused and then continued. "The CT-scan also detected a nodule in the bone on the fifth vertebrae in your back, near the spinal cord." *What? A tumor in Chris' back? Oh God.*

"We need to get an MRI to learn more about it and get control of it because if this tumor continues to grow, it could compress the spinal cord and possibly cause paralysis."

Neither of us could say anything. I struggled to breathe, feeling the weight of the news bearing down on my shoulders as if it was trying to crush me through the chair, onto the floor. The painful familiarity made me swallow hard in disbelief and my heart began to pound.

"I've already talked to the radiation oncologists and I want you to make an appointment right away. In the meantime, let's get an MRI to find out more about this tumor," Dr. Needles said and gave me the paperwork. The test was scheduled for the following week and we couldn't get in to see the radiologist until a week after the test. Two weeks of waiting.

Unable to find my voice, I squeezed Chris' hand, but he didn't say anything. Dr. Needles told us that he would look into another chemo regimen and encouraged us to hang in there.

While Chris drove home, I prayed for God to take my fear and to help me be there for my husband.

I'm not giving up, God. Show me what to do. Guide me in Your wisdom and strength to help Chris. You said, "Do not to be afraid." You are our God and You are with us. Hold us in Your loving embrace, carry us through this.

After saying this prayer, I felt a new sense of strength in my heart and I knew deep within me that God had already taken care of it. I wasn't afraid, I was confident. I wasn't lost, I'd been found in God's loving hands, in His amazing grace.

When we got home, Chris went to change his bandages and I took care of the dogs. I waited a long time before Chris finally opened the door slowly. I searched his eyes and felt fear at what I saw in them – defeat and sadness. I grabbed my husband and hugged him. A stream of tear drops fell on my shoulders while Chris held me tightly – as if his life depended on it.

"Steph, I am so scared." I held my breath, hearing the tremble in his voice. "I really don't know if I can handle being paralyzed. You know it's not living for me if I can't walk, run," he paused, as the tears soaked my shirt, "to never be able to ride my bike again," he sobbed, "and to never be able to play with our children. Steph, this is too much for me. I don't think I can handle this!" His body shook in my arms.

Something took over inside of me and I cradled Chris' face in my hands to make sure he could see my eyes and hear me.

"Chris, I want you to listen to me carefully. This is not going to happen. You will *not* become paralyzed. Do you hear me? This cancer is not getting the best of you and it will not take away your mobility. You will get back on your bike someday. You will be able to play with our children the way you want to. You will not be paralyzed. It's not going to happen. Do you understand?" I shook his shoulders and continued, "So, I want you to get this out of your head. Believe with all of your heart and soul, with all of your faith, hope, and love that you will ride your bike again. Believe it Chris."

He hugged me for a long time. I prayed my words had gotten through to him.

"I don't know what I'd do without you," he whispered in my ear.

"Chris, I want you to say it," I demanded.

"I believe, Steph." I searched his eyes and saw a new spark in them. He was back in his race.

Chris wanted to work on one of his models to calm down and relax. Once I was sure he was downstairs, I stood under the hot water in the shower and cried another mountain of tears. It was a crucial, intense moment and I thanked God again for His strength and wisdom to be there for my husband in the way he needed me.

Later, I sent an e-mail update to our family and friends to ask them to stay strong in their faith for Chris' healing and to keep fighting with us.

A few days later, Kelly called and shared a scripture from John 11:4,

"This illness will not end in death; rather it is for God's glory and the Son of God will be glorified in it."

"Steph, *'this illness will not end in death,'*" she said excitedly. "I was praying for Chris and I was led to this scripture. I'm a believer. I know God will heal Chris on His time schedule. We just have to hold onto our faith that everything is possible with God. Bob, the kids, and I will pray for God to work through Dr. Needles and guide him in the right direction. Please keep believing. We love you."

I continued to be amazed at how God shows His love for us by working through others.

Teddie Momma strongly urged us to attend an evening service over Labor Day weekend at her church, thinking we needed to be there. We were uplifted by the songs of praise and a message about unwavering hope. After the service, several pastors of the assembly walked over to us. They already knew what we were going through and offered words of encouragement, faith, and hope for us. They circled around Chris and offered a healing prayer for him, within him, and over him. We were in awe of the experience and felt deeply moved by their words of faith. We fervently believed that God was working on Chris' victory over the cancer. Before we left, one of the pastors pulled Chris aside to invite him to come to their Healing School. There was a surreal sense of peace within us that I believed was God's mercy. That night was one of the best nights of sleep we had had in a long time.

After talking more about this experience, we realized that we needed to call upon our elders of the church to pray for us.

"If anyone is sick, let him call on the elders of the Church. They shall pray for him, anointing him with oil in the name of the Lord. The prayer said in faith will save the sick person; the Lord will raise him up and if he has committed any sins, he will be forgiven."

- James 5:14 – 15

We invited our pastor, Father Don for dinner one night and told him about the latest discovery.

"Chris, at one point in our lives, we do have to die," Father Don said, taking Chris' hand, "but I truly believe it's not your time. I believe you still have work to do for God and that is to be a witness for others in your fight against the cancer." Then Father took my hand and continued, "Don't you know that you are already witnesses?" He asked, nodding. "Yes. You are a witness to me and to many others who have shared with me how much you are touching their lives with your testimony. And Stephanie, I'm sure through your e-mail updates you are reaching out to many more people. I believe it is your time now to do what God has called you to do. The love you both feel and share for each other is an amazing thing to watch. The way you look and interact with one another shows how deeply you love each other. I know God's love is within your love," he told us, smiling

Father Don encouraged us to continue reflecting over healing scriptures and also to pray over faith scriptures so that we could stay strong through our fight and share our testimony in the way God wanted us to.

After he left, Chris and I talked the rest of the night about our conversation with the pastors at Teddie Momma's church and Father Don. It was as if God was telling us, *As long as you keep fighting, I will keep fighting for you.*

"The Good Fight of Faith"

"Live in faith and love, with endurance and gentleness. Fight the good fight of faith and win everlasting life to which you were called when you made the good profession of faith in the presence of so many witnesses."

- 1st Timothy 6:11 – 12

Chris and I believed this scripture was an affirmation of what Father Don told us. We renewed our promise to stay strong in our faith, hope, and love. We agreed to keep moving forward and have a family, so I continued with my injections, medications, blood work, and ultrasounds.

By the second week of September, we met with a different radiation oncologist, Dr. Mackenzie, an average-height man with a lot of freckles. We bonded with his optimism and great sense of humor. He asked Chris to share his story and took notes. He told us that the nodule in the vertebrae was definitely a tumor about the size of a golf ball. Dr. Mackenzie was surprised to hear Chris hadn't experienced any backaches or pain.

"That's very good news, considering the size of the tumor. I'm sure you were shocked when you found this out. Unfortunately this is common with many cancer patients, but it is treatable through radiation," Dr. Mackenzie explained. My heart sank with the fear and agony that my husband would have to endure more radiation.

"Doctor, what kind of side effects should we expect from the radiation beams?" I asked nervously. Chris held my hand.

"The tumor is deeper in the body, so you may have redness or a dark spot and dry skin which are easily treatable." I took a deep breath, feeling relieved that Chris wouldn't have any more pain. "I suggest trying this for 10 days and go from there."

"Let's get started," Chris said. He met with the technicians to get tattooed and was told he could begin the treatment at the end of the week. I gave my fear about the radiation to God. I wasn't going to allow it to attack my mind and my heart. I knew God had already taken care of this and Chris would be fine.

After the third day of radiation treatment, we met with Dr. Needles to find out what else we could to do to fight the cancer. He wanted to try Methotrexate again by itself once a week for the next five weeks. However the insurance company wouldn't approve it since we had already tried it in 2007. Nancy, who had been our advocate for three years to get approval for all the treatments, told me what I needed to do while she continued to work on our behalf. Once I got home, I got on the phone and talked to anyone who would listen. After hearing the fourth person express their empathy and apologies about being unable to help us, I broke down. I was at a loss on what I could do to help my husband. Chris came up behind me, put his arms around my waist and hugged me tightly.

"Hey, it's going to be okay," he whispered. I leaned against his strong chest, realizing I had done it again – I let my emotions cloud over my faith. *When will I ever learn?*

"You're right, Chris. It's going to work out. God will make sure of it." I thought about the scripture from Isaiah 41:13.

"For I, Yahweh your God, take hold of your right hand and say to you, 'Fear not, I will help you.'"

A couple of days later, Nancy called Chris and told him to come in for the treatment, even though the insurance company still hadn't approved it. She promised that the bill would be taken care of. It had been over a month since the last chemo and Dr. Needles wanted him to get started sooner rather than later.

In the meantime, Chris was getting more excited about having a family. My doctor watched over me closely as I continued with the blood work and ultrasounds, constantly re-adjusting the dosage of my injections. All of these changes in my body made me irritable, impatient, and irrational. Just about anything set me off no matter how hard I tried to stay calm. By the end of September, I was so bloated that it was uncomfortable to walk, climb the stairs and stand up after sitting. Finally, I was ready to begin the IVF process and I couldn't stop smiling, hoping I would be pregnant soon. When I walked into the pre-op room, my doctor's eyes widened and she followed me into a room where Chris was helping me get on the bed.

"Stephanie, you look like you are in a lot of pain," she said. Surprised, I looked at Chris who was suddenly concerned.

"No," I shook my head, "No, I'm just very uncomfortable." She promised to get me ready as soon as possible and that I would feel relief afterwards. The next thing I knew, a nurse and an anesthesiologist came in and prepared me for the procedure. It felt strange to me that Chris was the one standing by the bed, holding my hand through all of this. When it was time, the nurse and Chris helped me walk to the surgery room. He wrapped his arm tightly around my waist.

"I love you, Steph. Thank you for doing this for us." I smiled at my husband and the next thing I knew, I was back in my bed again. It took some time to fully wake up and Chris was standing by my side, stroking my eyebrows.

"How do you feel?" he asked. I was about to answer when my doctor walked in, asking the same question.

"I feel good," I told them.

"I'm very happy to hear that, Stephanie. Everything went well, but I was getting nervous when I kept finding and retrieving one mature egg after another until I finally took the last one, totaling eighteen eggs altogether."

"Is that even normal?" I asked, shocked. She explained it was very unusual, but everything was fine. She told us the next step was to introduce Chris' "boys" to my "girls" and hopefully I would have a few embryos implanted by the end of the week. Chris was beaming with pride and kissed my cheek.

For a day, we didn't deal with cancer. We were a normal couple excited to start the family we had dreamt of, for so long. Everything possible was within our reach. All was right and well.

If only for a day.

Even though I felt sore, I returned to work the next day. I couldn't wait to find out how things were going at the fertility clinic. The minutes seemed to drag on, teasing me. I nearly jumped when I felt my cell phone vibrate in my pocket and saw that it was my doctor. Since I had students in my classroom, I found someone to cover for me and borrowed a colleague's office for privacy. When I called her back, I could tell by the tone in her voice that something was wrong. She asked how I was feeling and I told her that I was fine, although the trembling in my hands said I was lying. I gripped the phone so I wouldn't drop it and waited for her to tell me what was going on.

"We took the most mature eggs and introduced them to Chris' most active sperm and nothing happened." I took several deep breaths, trying to stay calm so I wouldn't miss anything she was telling me. "We tried again with the next best set, but there was still no success. We did a procedure to excite the sperm to make the tail-end of it curl up, which a few did and we tried again with the rest of your eggs, but nothing happened." She paused. In that dreaded moment of silence, everything stopped and was still. I knew what was coming next. I didn't want to hear it. *Oh God, could you take your remote control and pause the world for a few seconds for me?*

"I'm so sorry, Stephanie, but there is no possible way you and Chris can have a baby together."

Suddenly my hope and dream to bear Chris' children vanished like smoke disappearing in the air. You could never get it back and you will never see it again. It was gone... forever. From that smoke, a fire lit up inside of me. I sprung out of the chair and paced around in the empty office. I pulled at my hair wanting to feel any other pain than what I was feeling at that moment. *How much more can we take, God? Couldn't we just get a break from bad news? Why can't we have a baby together? It's not fair, it's not right! We live each day as best as we can, staying strong in our faith, hope, and love without giving up. Why Lord? Why?*

Feeling completely spent, I fell in the chair and sobbed on the desk. *I'm so sorry, God. I'm so sorry. But I'm so sad. I'm so angry. I'm so heartbroken. And I'm so confused.* I didn't know what to do except cry my mountain. *Oh God, how am I going to tell Chris? As much as I need Your help right now, how can I help my husband through this? Show me what I can do, what to say to him.*

I called my school nurse who knew what I had been going through and told her the news. She worked with my principal to find someone to finish the rest of the day for me so I could go home and be with Chris.

When I walked into the living room, it was as if Chris already knew, looking somber and stretching his hand out to me. We comforted each other through our tears, cradling each other in our sorrow over our lost dream. Neither of us could find any words. We couldn't say, "It's going to be okay," or "No worries." We sat for a long, long time. I prayed to feel God's love through our pain.

"Do you remember when we first met?" Chris asked breaking the silence. We shared our favorite moments: when we first held hands and couldn't tell whose hand was whose, that special kiss in the gazebo, when we expressed our love for one another, Chris' proposal, when we shared our wedding vows, the moment we became one, and the many moments of sweet expressions in our interactions, hugs, holding hands, and from our glances. We reminded each other of our love and God's love for us in everything we had gone through and would go through. So, to keep riding on in this race, Chris and I agreed to *"let love be in all"* of the journey.

- 1st Corinthians 16:14

Let Jesus' love embrace you. Let love be in your joy and laughter. Let love calm you with peace and contentment. Let love comfort your sorrows. Let love overrule hurt and heal your wounds. Let love forgive others who have wronged you. Let love surpass understanding and trust God. Let love build your faith. Let love be merciful to mend your heart. Let love be empathetic and compassionate. Let love be in the encouragement of your words and actions. Let love be in the gentleness of God's grace within you. Let love be your strength and courage to keep riding on. Let love be hopeful and bright like the colors of the rainbow. Let love be in simple, everyday experiences that take your breath away. Let love be the twinkle in your eye as bright as the stars at night. Let love be in hugs and holding hands. Let love be in your heart that comes out with a smile on your lips. Let God's love overwhelm you. *"Let love be in all."*

I couldn't understand why we had to go through so many obstacles in this race, but I knew God was with us in every part of it and He loved us very much.

"Do not be surprised at the painful trial you are suffering, as though something strange is happening to you. But, rejoice that you are in the very thick of what Christ experienced. This is a spiritual refining process so that you may be overjoyed when His glory is revealed" [to you].

- 1st Peter 4:12 – 13

I would keep riding on next to my husband, trusting my faith in God without ever giving up hope. I thanked God again for bringing Christopher Nicolas Saulet into my life and I couldn't wait to celebrate his birthday that was the next day.

I woke Chris up singing "Happy Birthday" and kissed him 50 times all over his face, making him laugh. I wanted to take the day off, but Chris insisted that I go to work since he had to go to the cancer center anyway for the third round of chemo. On the way to school, I asked God to bless Chris with a special and happy day.

When I got home, I found Chris relaxed and smiling in the living room. He described how the nurses in the chemo treatment room surprised him by singing "Happy Birthday" and gave him balloons tied to a gift bag filled with Butterfingers and Smarties along with some gag gifts. He smiled coyly.

"I'm not supposed to tell you, but one of the nurses gave me a kiss on my cheek." He looked so happy and I was thrilled that he had a good day. Chris was a little tired from the chemo so we stayed in and I made him a special birthday dinner. We turned in early and before falling asleep I sang "Happy Birthday" to my husband who fell asleep smiling.

Over the past several weeks, I had been secretly planning a surprise party for Chris. It couldn't have come at a better time for the both of us as I was getting more anxious over the final preparations. He decided to take a short road trip to Kansas City for a model show and I made him promise to be home by six – no questions asked. But I was the one who was surprised when Chris came home an hour early. I met him at the driver's side of the car with my hands on my hips.

"You're home early," I exclaimed.

"Is that a problem?" he asked, looking flabbergasted.

"Today it is," I answered, laughing.

"Geez, a guy just can't do anything right with his wife," he said, throwing up his hands.

"Chris, I'm trying to give you a surprise party and people are coming at six o'clock," I explained. Shocked he walked in the house and saw the decorations, but didn't say anything. I watched him sit down slowly on the window seat in our bedroom, combed his hands through his hair and took several deep breaths.

"I'm sorry I snapped. I just need to take it easy after driving so much and being at the show." I had never seen him so anxious and I didn't know what to do for him. I prayed to God to help relieve his anxiety. Chris deserved a celebration and I wanted him to have a great party.

"It's okay. Why don't we take things one at a time?" He nodded and started to relax a little. He wanted to change his bandages and clean up. I suggested taking an Ativan to help calm his nerves and he easily agreed, which surprised me because usually he would try to calm himself before resorting to a pill to do it for him.

It was over an hour before Chris was ready to join his party. I led him out into the backyard where everyone shouted *"Surprise!"*

"Oh wow," Chris exclaimed with a big smile, looking around. He stepped back, bowed his head, squinted his eyes, and pressed his lips together. After a few seconds, he went up to each person and thanked them for being there. Suddenly he saw Mark and Toni walking toward him. Chris raised his hands and let out a happy yell, hugging his oldest brother and sister-in-law. Chris didn't have much of a chance to catch his breath when he felt a tap on his shoulder and he slowly turned around to find his youngest brother smiling at him.

"Oh Michael," he cried as they greeted each other in a long hug. They stood side by side with their hands on their hips and nodding as they talked. They looked so much alike that they could easily have passed for twins.

Then Chris saw Bob several feet away and he made his way over to him. He stretched out his arms to embrace his best friend. They were more than friends, more than colleagues, more than cyclists – they were also brothers.

He looked around at our families, neighbors, and friends.

"Thank you," he choked. "I'm deeply touched you're all here with me and I am so happy at this moment." I stood by my husband and held his hand while he wiped his eyes. He squeezed my hand and I knew he was okay, but I kept a close eye on him as he visited with everyone and enjoyed his party with the gag gifts and funny stories.

We all learned more about Chris' mischievous side when Mark and Toni shared how he and some of his buddies formed the P.I.E. group. The letters stood for "Pie in the Eye" in which they planned out missions to throw a whipped cream pie at someone's face as a joke to one of their friends. Chris was the PIE man since he was the fastest runner in the group. He would throw the pie at the person and then take off like a flying bullet. They never got caught since they planned carefully and of course, hid their identity with ski masks. I looked at my husband, shocked, but then again, after all of the jokes he played on me, I shouldn't have been so surprised.

When we sang *"Happy Birthday,"* Chris blew out all 50 candles by himself.

"Thank you for being here to celebrate my birthday. This is the second time I had a birthday party with the people I cared about. I'm fortunate to have done so many things that I'm proud of during my 50 years. And even though I have cancer right now, it doesn't have me. I'm going to beat it and I plan on living another 50 years. And when I'm 100-years-old, I will still be riding my bike," he said confidently.

"If anyone can do it Chris, you can. And we'll support you all the way," one of our neighbors shouted and everyone cheered for him.

Chris was still on cloud nine as the party began to wind down, talking and laughing with his friends and family. Whenever I checked on him, he'd tell me he was fine except his cheeks were getting sore. During these priceless moments, I found myself wishing for time to tick slower or for more of it so we could savor it longer.

Looking back on that wonderful evening with our families and friends, I truly believe the love, support, and encouragement Chris felt from them gave him more courage to keep riding on in his race. Once again, God put the right people in the right place to say the right things to help us keep pedaling on.

About a week later, Chris woke up in the middle of the night with painful bladder spasms again. I wanted to take him to the E.R., but he didn't want to go.

"I've had enough of the E.R., Steph. If you'll help me, I think I can resolve the problem myself," he said, determined. I followed his directions while he slowly deflated the balloon, took his time to remove the catheter tube from his body and then inserted a new one, and finally inflated the balloon. It was a very long process and I became more amazed at his mentality, patience, and strength through each step. During a break, when he needed to relax, I teased him about finding a sexy nurse outfit.

"Woohoo!" he exclaimed, raising his eyebrows and laughing.

By the time he finished, the spasms subsided. He was so tired, he fell right back to sleep while I stayed awake and watched over him.

One evening, I heard Chris coughing in the bathroom and went to check on him. He couldn't stop and gasped for air. I massaged his back but he pushed my hand away and suddenly he stopped coughing and took a deep breath. He pointed to a small, round red phlegm floating in the toilet. Neither of us knew what it was and I hoped it wasn't anything serious. A few days later, Chris yelled out for me from the bedroom and I ran in to find him struggling to breathe and already panicking. I quickly found a small paper bag and held it to his mouth. I coached him to take long deep breaths until he was able to breathe calmly again. He sat down on the bed, trembling uncontrollably.

Realizing he wasn't cold, I immediately gave him an Ativan and massaged his back until his body finally relaxed and he was breathing normally again.

"I'm okay now, thanks," he said hoarsely, patting my leg. He told me that he started to feel warm from the lights while changing his bandages and then he couldn't catch his breath. When he tried to calm down, it got worse and that was when he called for me. I offered to call Dr. Needles' exchange but Chris insisted he was fine and we would be seeing him anyway the next day. I stayed awake again and watched my husband's chest rise and fall in a steady rhythm. I carefully rested my hand over his heart to feel the strong beats and prayed again for God's supernatural healing.

Dr. Needles scrunched his eyebrows together and shook his head after hearing about Chris' coughing spell and the breathing attack. He rested his elbows on his knees and bent closer toward my husband.

"One of the tumors in the lungs is wrapped around an artery," Dr. Needles said. "It's probably what's causing the coughing and breathing attacks. If it erodes," he paused, looking down at the floor and then back up at Chris, "it'll cause massive bleeding and there won't be anything we can do to stop it."

Oh... my... God! I sat there, staring at Dr. Needles, stunned.

"Doctor," Chris cleared his throat, "I'm not letting the cancer get the best of me. I'm going to keep fighting it, no matter what it takes." I looked at my husband with wide eyes.

"Okay Chris. Let's do the last round of the Methotrexate. We'll see what the CT-scan shows and go from there," Dr. Needles suggested. Watching them, I realized they were a good match for each other, fighting the good fight of faith and refusing to give up hope. I remembered when Chris told me he had chosen the right doctor, but I've since come to believe it was God who picked the right doctor for Chris, one who would keep riding on with him in his race.

Riding On

"Ride majestically! Ride triumphantly! Ride on the side of truth! Ride for the righteous meek!

- Psalm 45:4

For the next week, Chris didn't have any more coughing spells or breathing attacks, which made it easier on me to be at work for the first quarter conferences with my students' parents. Every chance I could, I called Chris to check on him and he'd laugh, assuring me he was fine.

During the third week of October, we met with Dr. Needles to find out the results of the CT-scan. As we waited patiently, we watched him study his notes.

"The cancer has gotten worse in the lungs. There are multiple new tumors – too many to count – in both lungs," he said.

Oh God, help us!

Dr. Needles cleared his throat and focused on Chris. "If you're interested, I have another chemo regimen in mind."

Chris nodded.

"We'll use Adriamycin, which we tried in 2007, with Cytoxan once every three weeks. The day after each treatment, you'll get a Neulasta injection and take medication to reduce nausea. We'll start with three rounds and then go from there."

"Okay, let's do it," Chris said and took the orders from Dr. Needles.

I took care of the co-pay and scheduled the next two rounds while Chris went into the treatment room. My mind was reeling over all that Chris had been through the past three years of his fight.

He endured 11 chemo regimens with 18 different drugs – four of them were repeated at least once – and two radiation treatments. This cancer was terribly evil and merciless. But it couldn't deter Chris' optimism, determination, humor, faith, hope, and love. He trusted God for healing and strength to ride on in his race. Even though this cancer kept attacking my husband, I deeply believed God would put it in its place – back to hell where it belonged.

After Chris was settled and the chemo was already pumping into his body, I watched him drift off to sleep. I pulled out my Bible and was

210

inspired to reread the scripture from Isaiah 41:11 and prayed over it while Chris slept through the treatment.

"Surely, all who rage against you will be put to shame and disgrace, all who fight against you will perish and come to nothing."

Later on that night, I shared those amazing words to Chris and we prayed again that this chemo regimen would fight against the cancer.

"Are you afraid?" I asked Chris softly. He shook his head firmly.

"No. I'm more determined than ever to keep on fighting and I feel stronger in my faith that God is helping me through it," he said confidently.

Chris continued to live each day as well as he could without letting the chemo get to him. He drove himself back to the cancer center the next day for the Neulasta injection, continued working on his models, stretched and exercised every day, and did chores and errands for me.

Chris was doing so well that he wanted to make a short trip to re-unite with some old friends, the Clark family. After Chris' mother re-married, he wanted to live with his oldest brother while finishing the last two years of high school before joining the Navy. It was during this time that Chris truly learned what it was like to be part of a family through the unconditional love from Mark and Toni and the Clarks. Chris met David Clark on the first day of school and they became good friends right away. David's family immediately accepted Chris and included him on many of their activities.

When we arrived at the restaurant, I was overwhelmed by so many people crowding around the doorway with barely enough room for us to walk through. One by one, they hugged Chris and then pulled me in their arms. I was deeply touched to see how much they cared and loved him. Throughout the evening, they reminisced over stories, jokes, and the fun times they had from their high school days.

When Chris was asked how he was doing, he expressed his faith about fighting against the cancer and his hope that he would be healed. Everyone offered encouragement, support through prayers, and optimism for him. It became another one of those pivotal moments at a time when Chris needed it the most and he was rejuvenated to keep on going. I shivered with goose bumps listening to their conversation and kept thanking God for getting us there.

By the beginning of November, which was during the third week of rest, Chris continued to deal with the spasms, throbbing pain from the scrotum, and discomfort from the creases. As the air was getting cooler, he struggled to catch his breath and would have more coughing spells at night.

I had hoped the problems would subside after the second round of the chemo, but Chris continued to struggle through them. Chris took each day and night one at a time, without complaining. He asked for home health care services again to help ease the pain in the creases and was approved for it. Chris had the same nurse who helped him heal from the radiation burns and was so happy to see her again. She offered different materials for bandaging and ointments to loosen the skin since it had gotten tight, causing the pain and limited flexibility and mobility.

As the Thanksgiving holiday quickly approached, Chris insisted on having dinner at our house with Mark and Toni and my family. I wasn't sure if it would be a good idea, thinking it might be too much for him. But I needn't have worried because he woke up with no pain and was in a great mood. He helped me prepare the two turkeys, while impersonating what he thought would be a turkey's voice, weaving a story about how they were innocently strutting around when they were captured, and then complaining about being stuffed. It had been a long time since we cooked in the kitchen together and it brought back so many memories when we carved a pumpkin, baked cookies, and made special meals together.

Chris had some time to rest before our house became crowded. The kids were running around and the kitchen was busy with the final preparations. We watched our families enjoy the meal together and I felt Chris squeeze my hand.

"Thanks for doing this, Steph. I'm so happy right now," he whispered, smiling.

A couple of days later, we met Dr. Chehval at the surgery center early in the morning for a cystoscopy to check Chris' bladder to find out what was causing the spasms. Afterwards, Dr. Chehval met me in the waiting room.

"Chris is doing well and is in the recovery room. The bladder is very irritated from the suprapubic catheter. We'll try a different prescription to calm the spasms," he said, patting my hand.

We continued to be hopeful that this chemo was working against the cancer and we had a lot to look forward to this Christmas.

December started out with Chris retiring from the Missouri State Highway Patrol after 25 years of service. He was so excited that he even felt up to going out to dinner to celebrate his accomplishment.

Two days later, Chris completed the last round of the chemo, but he was still having a lot of pain. Dr. Needles re-adjusted the pain medication and by the evening, it subsided. However, the winter air made it difficult for Chris to breathe and he started having more coughing spells. But Chris continued believing God was answering his prayers.

The end of the second week of December, another round of painful spasms woke Chris up and we worked together to flush the catheter tube until it cleared. Even though he was worn out, he still wanted to go to the annual Christmas party with Bob's family and see everyone again. Even though it was hard for Chris to tolerate the cold air, it was worth it to see the happiness in his eyes, talking and joking with our friends, watching Santa Claus pass out the gifts to the kids, and visiting with Grandma and Grandpa Schoonover. It turned out to be a great afternoon.

Driving home, I prayed that the party wasn't too much for Chris, but he was relaxed and content in the passenger seat, watching me.

"Thanks for helping me today. I'm really glad I went," he said, smiling sweetly.

"Me too," I choked, fighting the lump that already formed in my throat.

Several days later, Chris woke up early feeling pressure in his bladder. He tried to flush it out but couldn't clear the blockage. He didn't have an extra catheter tube to replace it, so we had to see Dr. Chehval who took care of Chris right away. I wondered how much longer Chris would have to deal with the catheter. Two years of the constant bladder spasms, blockage, and changing the tube every other week would make anyone want to say, "Enough! I can't take this anymore." But Chris just kept riding on.

We had planned to attend a support group meeting that morning and I didn't think Chris would want to go after the catheter problem, but he was excited to take me. The early morning snow caused problems on the roads and there was a lot of traffic. Chris insisted that he wasn't going to let the weather stop us and drove easily, without any problems. When he pulled into the snow-covered parking lot, he had a difficult time changing the gear to drive in it.

"Why can't I get this in the right gear?" he yelled breathlessly, gasping for air. Afraid he was going to have another anxiety attack, I calmly helped Chris control his breathing again. After several long minutes, his body calmed down. He put the car in the right gear and drove it into a parking spot. He sat there and closed his eyes. I wondered if it would be worth it for Chris to get out into the cold air again.

"I've had enough for today. Let's just go home," he said sadly. Suddenly I felt a strong intuition that we need to be at this meeting.

"Chris, I don't know why or how I know this, but we're supposed to be here. We've gone through so much this morning not to go inside and I'm not about to let you sit here defeated. We can do this Chris – together. Now, get out of the car."

Surprisingly, he obeyed and I met him just as he slid out of the driver's seat. I covered his mouth with a scarf and held him close to me, taking one slow step at a time, stopping often so he could catch his breath. After about 50 feet which was 15 minutes later, we finally reached the room. We were more than an hour late and I hoped that I didn't put him through this for nothing.

When we walked in the room, the pastor greeted Chris, throwing his hands up in the air and thanking God he was there. We started to apologize for being so late, but he shook his head.

"It doesn't matter, you were meant to be here at this moment," he told us. Chris and I looked at each other stunned.

"Thank you for getting me in here Steph," he whispered and kissed me.

The pastor began to read Ephesians 6:10 – 18.

"Be strong in the Lord with His energy and strength. Put on the whole armor of God to be able to resist the cunning of the devil. Our battle is not against human forces but against the rulers and authorities and their dark powers that govern this world. We are struggling against the spirits and supernatural forces of evil. This is no afternoon athletic contest that we'll walk away from and forget about in a couple of hours. This is for keeps, a life-or-death fight to the finish against the devil and all his angels. Be prepared! You're up against far more than you can handle on your own. Take all the help you can get. Put on the whole armor of God, that in the evil day, you may resist and stand your ground, making use of all your weapons God has issued. Take truth as your belt, justice as your breastplate, and zeal as your shoes to

214

propagate the Gospel of peace. Always hold in your hand the shield of faith to repel the flaming arrows of the devil. Finally, use the helmet of salvation and the sword of the Spirit, that is, the Word of God. Pray at all times as the Spirit inspires you. Pray long and hard. Pray for your brothers and sisters. Keep your eyes open. Keep each other's spirits up so that no one falls behind or drops out."

We were meant to hear this scripture and the pastor's teaching on it to use all that God gave us to fight the cancer. "Put on the whole armor of God" resembles getting dressed for a fight just as an athlete would put on what he needs to persevere through his race and cross the finish line. We learned to dress ourselves by getting into God's Word and grow from it, to deepen our relationship with Him and follow His lead, to share His truth with others through our faith, hope, and love, and to always pray. Chris and I felt a new sense of strength from this scripture – from God – to keep riding on side-by-side in our race.

The next day, I came home from school and found Chris sitting on the couch looking very serious. I stopped in the middle of my sentence as he stretched his hand out to me.

"Steph, everything is okay. I don't want you to worry." Confused, I sat next to him. "I called Dr. Needles and scheduled an appointment with him tomorrow afternoon. I know we were supposed to meet with him next week, but I need to talk to him about how to deal with the cold air and my struggle with breathing."

This was the first time Chris had ever requested to see Dr. Needles. The familiar pang of panic started to build up in my chest and I shook it away. Chris asked me not to worry, so I turned to God and leaned on Him for the strength I would need so Chris could lean on me.

"He is their strength in the time of trouble. And the Lord shall help them and deliver them."

- Psalm 37:39, 40

When we arrived at the cancer center, Chris struggled to catch his breath walking in from the parking lot.

"Do you want a wheelchair?" I asked nervously. At the beginning of the year when Chris had a difficult time moving around from the radiation burns, he rebuked me for offering a wheelchair and told me to never ask him that again. But this time, he accepted it and was grateful to sit down.

215

When I signed Chris in, several staff members were surprised to see him in a wheelchair. But he made good use of it with jokes, making everyone laugh.

When we got settled in a room, Chris rested his head in his hand and smiled sweetly. He looked so worn out, so fragile, so weak. I remembered the cancer patients I saw the first time we walked into the chemo treatment room. Chris was one of them. My heart throbbed painfully while I fought the tears that threatened and at the same time chiding myself to get a grip. The door slowly opened with Dr. Needles looking as sad as I felt and I wondered if someone had prepared him before seeing us.

"How are you doing, Chris?"

He told him about the panic attack and his struggle to breathe while Dr. Needles nodded, pressing his lips tightly. He pulled out his stethoscope, listened to Chris' lungs, and paused for several long seconds.

"Your lungs sound clear, but it seems that the cancer has gotten worse." He sighed. "I would like to do a chest X-ray to find out what's going on."

"What about the CT-scan and the MRI next week?" I asked.

"It will be better for Chris to have the X-ray," he explained and focused on Chris. "You can get it right away without having to make an extra trip. I know getting here today must have been difficult for you." Chris nodded slowly while I clenched my jaws to maintain some kind of control. "I also want you to take a breathing test to see if you are getting enough oxygen in your lungs. If you're not, you'll be put on oxygen to help you breathe easier." Chris easily agreed and I realized this was what he hoped for. Dr. Needles turned to me, "Stephanie, if the cancer is getting worse, then we will need to discuss hospice care for Chris," he said.

I felt dizzy as if the words were actual blows. I pressed my body against the back of the chair, trying to absorb the doctor's meaning. I couldn't find my voice and just nodded. He called to set up the chest X-ray and had one of the nurses take Chris for me. When I scheduled our appointment, I realized this could be our last meeting here. Trembling, I struggled to write it down, asking the receptionist several times to repeat it to me. When our eyes met, I lost it, shaking uncontrollably as the tears flowed down my cheeks. She immediately came around the desk and held me.

216

"Stephanie, there is always hope," she whispered. "Don't ever forget that."

I took several deep breaths to calm down and thanked her for all the times she encouraged us in our fight. When I came out into the waiting area, Chris was already back and found out he needed oxygen support. I looked at my husband with such wonder at how he could be so calm through all of this. I, on the other hand, felt horrible because I had let him down by being weak. But he smiled sweetly again and wiped away my tears.

Once Chris started getting oxygen, he began to breathe easily and started to relax. We were told that someone would come to our house later with more oxygen tanks and supplies. As we were leaving, we found out the temperature had significantly dropped causing the rain to turn to sleet. We needed to get home and Chris insisted on driving. I started to argue but the tone in his voice told me I already lost. I helped him climb in the driver's seat with the oxygen tank and gave him my keys.

I watched the tiny droplets hit the window, feeling physically, mentally, and emotionally drained. The last two hours felt like I've been going nonstop for two days and I couldn't grasp what was happening to us. What does hospice care mean for Chris? Does it mean no more chemo? Does it mean that there is no hope of beating the cancer? Does it mean that Chris is going to…? I shivered at the worse, feeling the cold of the weather seep in my bones and I realized we were already home as Chris slowly drove in the garage. I shook those thoughts away and focused on helping my husband get into the house. Chris wanted to sit on the couch for awhile. After he was settled in, he patted the empty spot and I snuggled close to him.

"Steph, I need you to believe that it's going to be okay," he said. He tilted my head to look at him. "I need you to say it."

"It's going to be okay Chris," I said.

"That's my girl," he smiled.

Later that night, Chris couldn't get comfortable in our bed and wanted to sleep sitting on the couch. I camped out on the other couch to be near him. Lying there, I thought of all that we had been through since we met. It seemed so long ago rather than four-and-a-half years. We finally found one another – Chris had waited much longer than me – and I prayed to God not to take us apart. I couldn't imagine my life without him. He added so much more joy, laughter, and love within me.

I got on my hands and knees and prayed for God's supernatural healing over Chris, remembering that Chris told me it would be okay.

Throughout the night, I would doze off only to be startled awake at the slightest noise. Several times I couldn't tell if Chris was breathing and I'd hold my own breath, until I saw his chest moving rhythmically. I thanked God again and tried to calm down to go back to sleep. It was one of those nights that seemed to drag on and on.

The next day was the last day of school before the winter break. It was a half-day with the students and the afternoon was free for the teachers to complete the report cards and prepare for the new semester. I almost didn't go, but Chris insisted he was much better and I should get my work done so I didn't have to do any of it during the holiday. I battled over leaving Chris and tried not to worry. I called every chance I had to check on him and each time, he assured me he was fine.

By the time the kids eagerly left to start their winter vacation, I was barely hanging on. Rather than going to the staff luncheon, I went to talk to my school nurse to find out more about hospice care. She explained that hospice offered a lot of support to make the patient comfortable and peaceful at the end of their life.

Oh God!

I doubled over in the most excruciating pain I have ever felt in my heart, sobbing at the thought of losing my best friend, my husband. She let me cry as she held me tightly, praying over me.

"The Lord is close to the brokenhearted; He rescues those whose spirits are crushed."

- Psalm 34:18

Finally, I pulled myself together to go back to my classroom so I could finish my report cards and prepare my lesson plans for the first couple weeks of the new semester.

When I turned off the lights, I noticed the darkness casting a shadow over the desks and felt its despair. I had no idea what was going to happen next in our race. I locked my door and turned my back against the dreariness that reminded me of death. When I stepped out into the bright December sun, I knew deep within me God would help us ride on to a higher hope.

Higher Hope

"Some see a hopeless end, while others see an endless hope."
- Author Unknown

I realized I needed people to hold me up so I could be strong enough for Chris to lean on me during the meeting with Dr. Needles. Poppa Bob offered to drive us which Chris gladly accepted and Kelly promised to meet us at the cancer center.

That morning, Chris struggled walking from the house to the car. Poppa and I had to brace him to help him keep his balance and even with the oxygen, he still gasped for air. I felt the weight in my chest grow, seeing how much weaker my husband had gotten over the last four days.

Oh God, give us both the strength we need.

Poppa pulled up as close to the entrance of the cancer center as possible and I went to get a wheelchair for Chris. It wasn't so hard to help him out of the car since the chair was right there for him and I quickly pushed him into the warm building. I helped Chris get settled and our favorite receptionist from the radiology department came over with tears in her eyes and hugged Chris lovingly. I heard her tell him how much he inspired her and she would keep praying for him. It was more than I could take until I felt a firm squeeze on my shoulder from Poppa, giving me some of his strength to keep going.

When I signed in, I saw more empathetic expressions from many of the staff who had grown to love Chris. As Poppa pushed Chris down the hall, several of them hugged me and reminded me there was always hope. I fought to stay in control, fighting the threatening tears and the lump that was already forming in my throat. Fortunately, we didn't have to wait very long when Dr. Needles walked into the room followed by Kelly. I started to calm down, feeling her strong positive energy. Dr. Needles sat down across from Chris.

"How have you been doing over the last several days?" he asked. I noticed he didn't have Chris' thick file with him and then realized he didn't need it anymore.

Oh God, I don't know if I can handle this.

"Breathing has become easier since starting oxygen, but I feel more tired than normal," Chris admitted. Dr. Needles listened to Chris' lungs and sat back down. The silence in the small room made me feel claustrophobic. I tried to breathe steadily to keep my heart from racing. Dr. Needles looked down, took a deep breath, and finally faced Chris.

"The chest X-ray isn't good, Chris," he paused. "It shows the cancer is getting worse in both lungs. It has taken over three-fourths of your right lung and about a half of your left lung."

Oh my God!

I couldn't bear to look at Chris, fearing I'd break down.

"May I see the X-ray?" Chris asked. Dr. Needles pulled it up on the computer screen. Looking at a pair of lungs that lit up the screen in a bright, glowing light, I fought the panic in my chest. After several long minutes, Chris cleared his throat.

"Can I try a different chemo?" Chris asked.

"At this point, doing chemo would reverse the benefits of it fighting the cancer. You would suffer more from the side effects because your body can't take it anymore," Dr. Needles explained. Chris nodded, rubbing his chin thoughtfully.

"Can I do a lung transplant?" The unbearable pain in my heart grew watching my husband try to keep riding on in his fight, to find any other course that could lead him to the victory we've hoped for.

Dr. Needles patiently smiled and shook his head. I was on the verge of losing it and hugged my notebook as if it could somehow support me.

"What's the next step?" Chris asked.

"We would do hospice care, Chris," Dr. Needles answered and told us it would start later in the afternoon at home. We won't have to make any more trips to the cancer center. The hospice nurse would come to our house to care for Chris and offer the kind of support we would need. Dr. Needles would still be his doctor and the nurse would stay in constant communication with him.

"Even though you won't be doing any more treatment, there is always hope," Dr. Needles said. Chris nodded thoughtfully.

"Thank you for helping me in my fight," he said and they shook hands.

"Chris, you've been an inspiration," Dr. Needles responded.

Before we left, Chris wanted to see the nurses again in the chemo treatment room while several other staff members shared how much

Chris inspired them and they would keep him in their prayers. I struggled to keep the tears in control and excused myself to go to the bathroom. When I walked back in the waiting room, Kelly and Chris were laughing and fighting over sugar cookies.

"How many cookies have you eaten, Chris?" I asked, stunned.

"I'm not telling' cuz they're all for me," he answered with his mouth full.

"I don't know Chris," Kelly chimed in. "I've seen how many you took and when you're not looking, I'm going to take one."

"Oh no you won't," he challenged and hid them all under his sweatshirt.

When Poppa and I were helping Chris get in the car, he was still protecting his cookies.

"I promise, I won't take any of your cookies, Chris." Poppa told him.

"I know, but keep her away," he said pointing at Kelly. "I don't trust her around my sugar cookies." We all burst out laughing.

Later that night, after meeting with a case manager to begin hospice care, Chris and I talked for a long time. We agreed to give it all up to God and put it in His hands. No more doctors, lab work, tests, or treatments. God is an amazing God who can do awesome things for us. We renewed our vow to not give up.

"Let us hold fast to our hope without wavering, because He who promised is faithful!"

- Hebrews 10:23

"To hope is the way we are saved. But if we saw what we hoped for, there would no longer be hope. How can you hope for what is already seen? So, we hope for what we do not see and we will receive through patient hope."

- Romans 8:24 – 25

I called our families and sent out an e-mail update with the news.

Michael encouraged us to stay strong in our faith and hope, to keep praying, and to give our problems to God to handle for us. He asked us to re-read Romans 5:1 – 5 which tells us that we would be tested in our faith and teaches us how to deal with the test.

"One thing I know for sure is that God is not finished with His plan for Chris yet," Michael told me.

The next day was Christmas Eve and our house was in constant motion with people coming and going with medical supplies and medication. We had to change oxygen equipment because the hospice care used a different company and I had to relearn how to operate it while Chris adjusted to a new oxygen tube. To my surprise, it didn't bother him and he went along with all the changes in our home. By the time Carol came, I fell in her arms desperately needing my sister to hold me and give me strength.

"Shush, I'm here," she whispered, holding me tight.

She helped me understand how to monitor Chris' oxygen level and organize his medications in a way that didn't seem so overwhelming. I was beginning to feel more at ease when Chris' hospice nurse, Terry, arrived. I noticed the kindness in her light blue eyes and the friendliness in her smile right away. She took the time to get to know Chris, asking questions about himself and joking with him. I knew they were going to be a good match for each other just as Chris was with both of his doctors. When he was ready, he told her his story as she listened carefully, taking notes.

"I want you to know, I'm not giving up," Chris told her.

"There is always hope Chris," Terry said, nodding. She explained that her role was to help take care of him and offer both of us support. She asked other questions to find out more about his needs. She was surprised to hear how long he had dealt with a suprapubic catheter and was even more amazed to learn he could flush it out and replace it himself. When it was time to change his bandages, Chris felt comfortable enough to have Terry assist him. She carefully helped my husband up from the couch and walked with him to our bathroom. She encouraged me to take a break and promised to call me if they needed me. When I walked back into the dining room, Father Don was talking to Carol in the kitchen. I rushed over into his arms. He hugged me tightly while praying for Chris and me.

"How did we get here?" I asked them. "It's not supposed to happen this way. Chris was supposed to be cured from the cancer, not...." I couldn't say the three-letter word. I looked at my sister. "We couldn't be brought together only to share a short season of our lives." Carol dried the tears from my cheeks and stroked my hair like she used to do when I was a little girl.

"There is always hope," Father Don reminded me.

Even in the darkest of nights, there was a bright shining star, far beyond, in the black night sky, twinkling for us to follow its glorious light of hope. It was up to Chris and I to reach up toward that light with all of our love and this light would brighten our hope to keep riding on together.

When Chris and Terry walked into the dining room, he was thrilled to see Father Don.

"Hi Father," he smiled. "It's good to see you." Father Don stood up and hugged my husband. After Chris was settled on the couch again, Father Don spent time with him while Terry shared her evaluation of Chris in the dining room. Carol sat next to me and held my hand tightly as Terry explained how cancer would eventually take Chris' life. It was more than I could take, struggling to stay strong in my hope.

"Terry, he is not going to give up." I choked, trying to get my words out. Carol squeezed my hand again. "How can I tell my husband that he is dy... dy...?" I couldn't say the word. "How can I tell my husband that the hope he's hung onto and fought for is not the hope to heal him? To tell him these things is to tell him to give up. I *won't* do that to him."

She encouraged me to take things one day at a time and went over the paperwork we would go over at the end of each visit. She showed me how to document what medicine Chris took, the reason, and the time he took it. She also wanted me to monitor and record whenever he was in pain and the intensity of it so she could work with Dr. Needles to re-adjust the dosage. She emphasized that the goal of hospice care was to help Chris be comfortable and peaceful. I kept nodding while she talked, but I couldn't keep up or follow along anymore. I had reached my limit.

For more than three years, we had battled this cancer, and this was not the finish line we had hoped for. It couldn't end like this.

"The Lord is good for those who hope; in the day of trouble, He shelters them. He remembers those who trust in Him."

- Nahum 1:7

That night, after everyone left, I watched over my husband as he slept sitting on the couch again and let the tears flow freely.

Oh God, what can I do for Chris? How can I take his pain away? How can I make him feel better? Show me what to do to be there for him in every way he needs me? Help me to be strong for him. Only You can give me the strength, the courage, and the love to keep riding on with my husband.

Christmas Day was very quiet compared to the day before. Chris and I celebrated the amazing love that brought this special holiday. We prayed thanks to Jesus for His good news and His loving sacrifice for us, for bringing us together, and for healing in Chris' body. Chris slept most of the day as I stayed next to him on the couch. In the back of my mind, I wrestled and fought against the possibility that it could be our last Christmas together. I couldn't imagine my life without Chris. I shook my head at the thought of it, reminding myself that there was always hope and prayed to God for healing within Chris.

Later in the afternoon, Chris kept waking up from the stabbing pains in the scrotum. I tried to find different ways to position him to help him get comfortable. Every wince, cringe, and gasp of breath pulled on my heart. I prayed for guidance and wisdom to help my husband, and for God to take away his pain. Eventually Chris would fall back asleep when the pain medicine started working for him. I was anxious to see Terry the next day to find out what I could do to help Chris be more at ease and pain-free.

Once again, our house was in full swing with more deliveries. As Terry and I went through all of the supplies in the dining room, I learned more ways how to help Chris.

"Terry, have you talked to Dr. Chehval about draining the fluid in the scrotum? It is causing so much unbearable pain for Chris." I asked. She remained busy checking an item for several long seconds, and then finally looked at me.

"I don't want to be the one to have to tell you this, Stephanie, but you have the right to know." Confused, I shook my head. Terry sighed, "It's not fluid in the scrotum."

"Then what is it?" I asked, still not catching on to where she was going.

"Stephanie," she paused, "it's a tumor." For a moment, everything stopped.

"What? A tum... a tumor? Are you sure?" I asked, keeping my voice low so Chris couldn't hear me from the living room. She nodded. After all Chris had been through from the radiation – all of that pain, suffering and misery he endured. And throughout it all, a new tumor had grown?

"I need a minute," I whispered and stormed out the back door into the cold winter air, hoping it could cool the anger in my chest, threatening to explode. I paced back and forth in the middle of the yard, cursing at the cancer. I looked around at what I could hit and found nothing. I took one of our plastic chairs and threw it across the lawn. It wasn't enough. I grabbed another chair and threw it. Then I threw another one and another one until there was nothing else I could throw. I wanted to grab a hold of this cancer, pull it out of my husband's body, drench it in gasoline and burn it back to hell where it belonged. The knot in my stomach made me heave and I crouched over in so much pain – the worse pain I have ever felt in my life. I straightened myself up and raised my arms toward the Heavens with tears streaming down my face. *God, oh God, have mercy on my husband! Give me the strength I need for him.*

I stood there, looking at the clouds and suddenly realized that I must give Chris up to God completely with all of my faith and trust, hope, and love. As much as I didn't want to let go of my best friend who was the love of my life, I knew he belonged to God, not to me. How could I let him go? *God forgive me, but I don't want to let him go – I want him whole again, healthy and strong. I want to go back when we were dating and stay there frozen in time. Oh God, how can I get through this? How can I help my husband through this?*

I have no idea how long I was outside. Slowly, I picked up all the chairs, feeling physically, mentally, and emotionally drained, but somehow I felt strong. I didn't understand it, but I held my head high and went inside to take care of my husband.

"He will uphold all those who fall and lift up all who are bowed down."

- Psalm 145:14

Terry was helping Chris change his bandages so I organized the materials and supplies. When she went over the paperwork, I talked with her about the tumor.

"Do not tell Chris that it's a tumor. Tell him the same thing the doctors told us – that it would risk infection to drain it or whatever you can ethically say about it," I begged. She twisted her pen and shook her head. "Please, Terry. You have no idea how much Chris suffered from that radiation. His wounds you see now are nothing compared to what they were during and after the treatment. It would crush him if he knew there is a tumor after all he went through."

I gasped for air, struggling to get the words out. "Terry, if he is to ask you if there is a tumor there, then you have to tell him. But he won't ask. So please, don't tell him. Don't let this man suffer any more than he already has. Please." She pressed her lips together, still shaking her head.

"Okay, Stephanie. But if he does ask if it is a tumor...,"

"Terry, he won't. I know my husband," I whispered. "Thank you."

Wondering if I was doing the right thing, I wrestled over not telling Chris about the tumor. I knew God was watching over us when Bob came by several days later. I was so happy to see him and realized he was the one I needed to talk to. After I told him, Bob was quiet for a long time.

"I think you're doing the right thing, but Stephanie, if he asks if it's a tumor then you need to tell him the truth," Bob said.

"Let's hope he doesn't ask, Bob," I whispered. He squeezed my hand and then went to hang out with his best friend.

Over New Year's, Patrick, Mark and Toni and their daughters came to visit us and met Terry. They began to understand what hospice care meant and cherished their time with Chris. It was good for Chris to see his family again, especially his nieces. They all brought a lot of laughter and energy to us and Chris smiled a lot, enjoying every moment of it. After a few days, they all had to go back to work, but Mark decided to stay a week with us. He spent a lot of time with Chris giving him foot massages, telling funny stories to make him laugh, and comforted him through his pain.

After Mark left, it was just Chris and me again. During some peaceful waking moments, we enjoyed just being together and grew deeper in love. Each night I'd thank God for giving us a day together and each morning I thanked Him for blessing us with a new day.

One late afternoon, after changing the bandages with Terry, Chris was very quiet when he came back to the living room. I knew something was wrong. When Terry reviewed the paperwork, she told me about their conversation in the bathroom.

"Stephanie, Chris asked me when I thought he would be able to get off the oxygen support." I held my breath, already knowing what she told him and I felt his agony in my heart.

"What did he say?" I asked.

"He was quiet and then he asked me if I thought he would ever get better again," she whispered sadly.

"What did you say to him?"

"I couldn't speak, I just shook my head. Chris didn't say anything else. I asked if he knew what this meant and he nodded once." Tears streamed down my face, feeling my heart break again for my husband. I buried my head in my hands, hurting so much for him. I prayed for

God to help Chris through his anguish. I prayed for wisdom and comfort for my husband. As I was wrestling to let him go, I was at a loss on how to help him through it.

Oh God, how did we get here after fighting so hard for so long?

I stayed close to Chris and he was quiet all night. I knew I had to wait until he was ready to talk to me about his conversation with Terry. The next morning, we were talking about movies and I was trying to get him to laugh. I teased him about watching a popular musical that was out at the time, hoping to get a funny reaction from him.

"You can watch it after I'm gone," he scowled. I held my breath, noticing the anger in his voice and lifeless eyes. He had never said those words before.

Oh God, is Chris giving up? Has he lost hope? I didn't know what to say or how I could comfort him. All I could do was stay by his side and hold his hand.

"Do you know what Terry said to me last night?" he asked, looking down, still avoiding my eyes.

"Steph, I asked her when I'd be able to get off the oxygen and she told me that I'll have it for the rest of my life." I squeezed his hand. "Do you know what this means, Steph? It means I will never be able to ride my bike again." I brought his hand to my lips.

"Chris, I am *so* sorry," I choked. "But you're not alone. I'm right here with you. I love you." He squeezed my hand and nodded, but he didn't say "I love you" back. It nearly broke me, sitting there feeling so lost and wondering where our hope is in all of this. Several hours later, I was barely hanging on when Carol came and I fell in her arms sobbing over what had happened. I didn't know what I could do to help my husband and I felt that I was losing him. Carol encouraged me to take a break and go to mass at my church while she stayed with Chris.

"I'll never forget the trouble, the utter lostness, the feeling of hitting the bottom. But there's one other thing I remember, and remembering, I keep a grip on hope. God's loyal love is created new every morning. I'm sticking with God. He's all I've got left. God proves to be good to the man who passionately waits, to the woman who diligently seeks. It's a good thing to quietly hope, quietly hope for help from God."

- Lamentations 3:19-26

During the service, I knew – deep within me – I was supposed to be there to talk to Father Chris, who was Father Don's assistant. I waited until everyone was gone to talk to him.

"Father, how do I help my husband through hospice while I'm trying to deal with it myself? How do we keep hoping?" He put his fists together and pressed them against each other.

"You and Chris have been fighting against this cancer, hoping for his healing a long time without ever giving up. Just like my fists here, pressing against each other without wavering, you both have been through so much pain and yet you stayed strong in your faith while loving each other through it all. Eventually the strength of my fists will grow weak and I'll begin to feel the pain flow in my knuckles, into my hands and wrists and through my arm until I finally release them." Father Chris let his fists go and opened up his hands.

"Sometimes when you have hoped for one thing for as long as you and Chris have for healing from this cancer, you get to a point when you have to let go for a much higher hope." I studied his hands, facing upward and began to understand what Father Chris was saying. "It's not giving up when you let go of one hope to open yourself to a much higher hope. Stephanie, for each one of us, the greatest hope of all is to live an everlasting life with Jesus Christ."

This was what I was supposed to hear and learn to help Chris. I thought a lot about what Father told me. I still didn't want to let go of my husband, but I knew I needed to do this for him, for us, and for God.

Chris was still in a solemn mood when I came home and I knew it wasn't the time to talk to him yet. Poppa Bob and Carol urged me to get some rest and promised to stay up with Chris. I laid in bed and prayed again for God's mercy, grace, wisdom, strength, and healing for the both of us. I prayed especially for my husband to come back to me so I could help him through this. I was falling asleep when suddenly I was startled awake and nearly scared Poppa and Carol, jumping out of bed to be by Chris' side at the doorway of our bedroom.

"Thank you, you can leave now," Chris told them. They left the room reluctantly, whispering apologies. I faced my husband and held my breath as I noticed life in those beautiful brown eyes. "I'm not giving up, Steph!" and he embraced me hard. I felt like Chris was back and thanked God for hearing my prayer. "I love you, Steph. I'm so happy you're in my life. I prayed for a woman like you, and God sent me an angel."

"God sent me a hero," I whispered, stroking his face. "I love you so much."

He wanted to try sleeping in our bed, so I helped him as gently as I could to get comfortable. I cuddled close to him and held his hand. It had been two weeks since we had slept next to each other and according to Carol and Poppa who checked in on us, we slept through the night.

Several days later, I knew it was time to talk to Chris about a higher hope. It was a rare time that we were completely alone. I had to look beyond myself and prayed to God for the words He wanted me to tell my husband. I felt a strong sense of peace within me that I couldn't understand, but I knew it was from God. Chris had just finished changing his bandages and was comfortably propped up against the pillows on the bed with a smile that made my heart skip a beat. I sat in front of him by his feet.

"Chris," I said softly. He looked at me with those eyes I adored. "We need to talk. You know how much I love you and I know you love me just as much. Even though we are going through all of this, I am still so happy with you."

Chris blew me a kiss and I blew one back to him.

"I'm very proud of the man you have become throughout your fight. You have shown such incredible strength, will, perseverance, optimism, humility, faith, and hope. Above all of this, you have shared your love with me, our families, and close friends. You have fought so hard for so long and I'll always be by your side to support you. But, Chris," I choked, "after awhile, your body starts to get tired and weak, even though your spirit is stronger than ever. It's like pressing my fists together and keeping them like this for a long time without wavering or letting go. Eventually my hands will become fatigued and I would feel pain travel through my fingers, hands, wrists and up into my arms. Even though I refuse to give up hope that I can keep my fists together, my physical body has endured so much that it has grown tired of keeping up with my spiritual will to keep pressing my fists together, still hoping and fighting strong. So, I have to come to terms that I have to let go of this kind of hope, open up to a higher hope, and release my fists from the fight." I opened my hands.

"Look at my hands, Chris. I'm not giving up on hope for your healing. But I am also looking beyond that hope to a much higher hope for you. This kind of hope is what we all have in our spirit, which is to be with Jesus once again – when we are ready, when it is our time. It's not giving up when you look above and beyond to be with Jesus. You are the strongest man I know to have gone through as much as you have over the past three years in your fight against the cancer. While it keeps attacking your body, it never could attack your faith, your hope, and your love. Chris, you *are* victorious over the cancer. I want you to know this, *believe* in it, with God on your side – this cancer cannot destroy your spirit. I love you so much more than my own life," I swallowed hard and took a deep breath, "and I want you to look beyond to the greatest hope of all – when you are ready – and I will let you go. I'll be okay, and I know you'll watch over me, that you will be *my* angel." I couldn't talk anymore.

Chris studied me intensely and then nodded one time.

"Okay," he said slowly and then paused for a long time, keeping his eyes on me. "But I'm not ready yet."

Even though Chris refused to give up on his fight, he continued to suffer unbearably. One day, I was helping him in a chair in the living room when he winced loudly. I asked what I could do to help him and he angrily snapped at me.

"There's nothing you can do!" Stunned, I was speechless while fighting back the tears. Terry immediately came to Chris' side and suggested I get a pain pill for him. Not knowing what to say, I followed her order and left the room. I looked out the kitchen window and did the only thing I could do, I prayed desperately. *God, there is only so much this man can take. Please help him. Show me what I can do for him to relieve his pain.*

When I came back, I saw Terry comforting my husband, holding his hand and encouraging him to agree to a morphine pump to help ease his pain. To my surprise, he easily accepted the idea. After she left, I stayed by Chris' side, hoping and praying he would get relief soon. When I looked up, there were large tears in the corner of his eyes. I wiped them away.

"I'm so sorry," he whispered.

"I love you, Chris. It's going to be okay. No worries."

I don't know where he got the strength, but he pulled me up toward him, kissed me, and hugged me tightly.

"I love you too, Steph."

During the last two weeks in January, the morphine pump was effectively managing Chris' pain and he kept on fighting even though his body was getting weaker to the point he had to use the wheelchair to get around the house. At first he balked at the idea of using one until

I called it a transport and he accepted it as long as he could walk a couple of feet from time-to-time. However, he did use the transport to his advantage.

One day, I was holding Chris' oxygen tube in front of him while Terry pushed him and he bumped my lower backside with his cane.

"Woohoo, sexy lady!" he exclaimed, smiling mischievously. Shocked I turned around to find him laughing and giving me a slow wink.

"You need to behave or else I'll find a way to pinch you on your bottom when you least expect it," I told him, pointing my finger and laughing. When I turned around, Chris bumped me again.

"Woohoo, I hope you do baby," he said.

His sense of humor didn't stop there. One day, Father Chris came by for a visit. Chris was eating Jelly Bellies and offered some to him.

"So, Father Chris," he started and paused for a long time. "How is God's business going?"

"Uh, did you ask me 'How is God's business going'?" Father asked, surprised. Chris bobbed his head in a yes motion.

"Yeah," he slurred. "How... is... God's business going?"

"Well, things are going well," he answered, laughing. Chris offered him another Jelly Belly and I left them alone to talk. After awhile, Father came out into the dining room and asked us to join them in the bedroom. Chris was starting to feel tired and I helped him lie back down in bed. Carol, Teddie Momma, Kelly and Father Chris joined hands in a circle around us. Chris closed his eyes listening to Father's prayer and our words of hope and love for him.

"Thank you," Chris whispered, smiling as he drifted off to sleep.

Chris kept on going even though Terry warned me that it wouldn't be long for him. The pain from the tumor and the struggle to breathe intensified so much Terry talked to Dr. Needles and he increased the dose. Chris began to sleep more and whenever he was alert, he was very slow at processing information and talking in conversations, but he still knew what was happening around him and he still kept riding on.

One day, Chris was enjoying a massage in the living room while I sat with Poppa Bob and Father Don in the dining room. The therapist came to join us to do her paperwork and told me Chris was completely relaxed and sleeping peacefully on the couch.

"What's happening, babe?" Chris asked. I turned around, stunned to find him standing in the doorway, leaning on his cane in front of him with a drunken grin on his face. It had been a week since he had been on his feet by himself. I got up to help him, but he shooed me away with his cane.

"I got it. It's all under control," he said and scooted several steps over so he could lean against the wall. He stood there like Charlie Chaplin balancing on the cane in front of him, smiling mischievously. I started to walk toward him and he pointed his cane at me.

"If you come closer, I'm gonna have to bump you on that sexy behind of yours again," he threatened, winking at me. I looked at the therapist, shocked.

"What have you done to my husband?" I asked, laughing.

Chris looked at everyone with a silly grin and then checked out his cane as if it was the first time he had ever seen it. He began to do a soft-shoe dance with it, humming a little tune to go with his steps. After several minutes of his show, he became quickly fatigued and he let me help him back to the living room.

Several days later, we had a house full of people: Poppa Bob, Momma Sue, Carol, Bob and Kelly with their kids, and some of our neighbors. We were sitting around the dining room table, talking and laughing at stories about Chris. He looked at everyone with a wide smile as he listened to Bob's jeers and jibes at him, shaking his head and rolling his eyes at his best friend. Then Bob got on a roll and told us "The Jackass" story.

"We were riding somewhere on a country two-line road, cruising at about 35 to 40 miles-per-hour. We had a momentum together and were enjoying a really nice ride until a redneck in a pick-up truck came up behind us, blasting his horn and yelling at us, barely missing Chris as he sped by. Chris yelled back at him, 'You jack-ass!' The guy screeched to a halt and got out of his truck. In one swift movement, Chris stopped, dropped his bike in the middle of the road, and threw off his helmet then walked toward the guy, yelling at him to get back in his truck. I'm standing there in shock and disbelief," Bob said.

"Then I thought, 'Oh my God, he just dropped his brand new bike in the middle of the road.' I couldn't believe it. I picked up his bike, made sure it was okay, and then picked up Chris' helmet. At this point, Chris and the guy were nose-to-nose, yelling at each other and I heard Chris call him a 'jack-ass' several more times. When I caught up with them, I was standing behind Chris, holding the two bikes up and agreeing with everything he said to the guy. All I kept saying was, 'Yeah, what he said. Yeah, yeah – that too.'

Finally the guy turned around and left and Chris shook his head. After we got back on our bikes, Chris cooled off.

Really, Chris, 'jack-ass?' I asked him, laughing. That's the best you could come up with? 'Jack-ass?' Chris gave me a dirty look, told me to shut up and keep riding."

Everyone burst out laughing while Chris nodded proudly. It felt like old times, enjoying our friends again. I looked over at my husband and our eyes met across the table. He winked and blew me a kiss. I felt a flutter in my stomach. Chris could still sweep me off my feet.

Later on, after we settled in bed for the night, Chris told me he had a really good time.

"It was so good to see everybody, Steph. I had fun tonight," he said, smiling as he fell asleep.

The next day, Mark and Patrick came. They walked in the bedroom quietly and suddenly Chris woke up as if he sensed their presence.

"Hey guys," he said weakly, reaching his hand out to shake theirs, smiling. He had been asleep all day, but he was able to stay alert long enough to talk them.

Michael came the following day and once again Chris woke up when he heard his brother's voice, but he couldn't keep his eyes open and fell back asleep. Chris slept a lot while we all took turns monitoring the morphine pump and worked together to change the bed sheets and clean him. I was deeply touched by the strong bond and love between Chris' brothers and thanked God they were here.

Terry held a family meeting about what to expect during Chris' last days. The heaviness of the pain bore down on my heart, listening to Terry's words. I couldn't stand to hear this over again and left to be with Chris. We weren't alone very long when Father Don slowly walked into our bedroom.

"May I join you," he asked and I smiled at him. He sat in the chair next to Chris and held his hand, talking to him with such loving and encouraging words. Tears streamed down my cheeks feeling the love this man had for Chris.

"How are *you* doing, Stephanie?" he asked.

"I'm doing the best I can for Chris," I answered.

"Stephanie, tell Chris about Heaven." I studied Father Don's encouraging eyes, scooted closer to Chris on the bed and began to tell him what I thought Heaven was like.

"Oh Chris, Heaven is an amazing place. Once there, you won't feel any pain. You'll feel so free and exhilarated and strong again. I bet you'll be reunited with your mother and then finally see Jesus. Imagine Chris, being in His presence?

The colors there are nothing like the colors we see here on Earth. They are so bright and full of love. Everything there has its own beautiful tune. For example the flowers actually sing to you. You can hear music from a waterfall. Everything is so glorious and beautiful in Heaven because everything and everyone is with God. There is so much love surrounding you that all you can do is embrace it and share it with others.

There are many rooms in Heaven and each one is as incredible as the other. Jesus told his disciples how he had to return to Heaven in order to prepare many rooms for us. The floors are the most beautiful marble you'll ever see, and the walls and columns are gold with the ceilings open to the Heavenly skies. You'll be able to explore Heaven and beyond, Chris. You can go to the moon, to the planets, and to another universe if you want.

You can get back on your bike and just ride on and on. Can you imagine riding your bike through the Heavens? Oh, Chris, you'll feel so free, so happy, and so loved in Heaven. Heaven is truly a much bigger hope for us. It's a place where we can be in the presence of Jesus forever. Chris, I want you to look forward to this kind of hope – I want you to go home to Jesus and be with Him in Heaven."

I couldn't speak anymore. As much as I didn't want my husband to die, as much as I wanted to be selfish to keep him in my life, I had to let him go. I loved this man and my God so much, I wanted Chris to be with Him again. I looked over at Father Don and he nodded, smiling at me. I watched him pray over Chris and bless him. Then he walked over to me, hugged me tightly. Rather than feeling exasperated, there was a sense of peace deep within me.

Heaven is an endless hope that is the highest hope for us all.

The Midnight Rally

"Our light and momentary troubles are achieving for us an eternal glory that far outweighs them all. So we fix our eyes not on what is seen, but what is unseen. For what is seen is temporary, but what is unseen is eternal."

— 2nd Corinthians 4:17-18

As we all got settled in for what we already knew was going to be another long night keeping up with the morphine pump for Chris, Carol and I were talking quietly by him.

"You both looked so happy in that picture," she said, looking at our wedding picture taken of us in the park. When I glanced at the photo, it seemed to me that it was such a long time ago instead of only two-and-a-half years since that wonderful day.

"Oh Chris, I love you so much," I whispered in his ear and kissed his cheek. Carol touched Chris' chest.

"Steph, he is so strong. I can't get over how strong his heart is. He took very good care of himself. He's fighting so hard." Then she turned to Chris, "Chris, you are so brave." I was deeply touched by the gentleness in my sister's voice and the loving care she gave to both of us over the last several days. I knew it hadn't been easy for her or on everyone else staying by our side — physically, mentally, and emotionally — but they endured it all to be there for us. There was so much love in our house. I silently thanked God for all of them.

"Chris, you have been very strong throughout this fight. I am so proud of you," I whispered and kissed his cheek. I held his hand and stayed close by him.

Mark soon came into the room with Poppa followed by Michael and Patrick. We were all very quiet, lost in our own thoughts, keeping watch over Chris. Even the air was still until a ring from Pat's cell phone broke the silence. Patrick left the room and suddenly I noticed Chris' eyes fluttered.

"Did I just see Chris blink his eyes?" I asked everyone, watching Chris. I sat up to face him and stroked his cheek, whispering his name over and over. Slowly, ever so slowly Chris blinked his eyes like he was beginning to wake up from a sound sleep. After a few minutes, it seemed like he was able to focus in on us and turned toward me as I called his name. His eyes lightened and he smiled sweetly, puckering his lips for a kiss. I moved the breathing tube out of his mouth into his nose and kissed him.

"I love you, Chris."

"Love... you," he mouthed and smiled again. He slowly turned his head over to his right and saw Carol who gave him encouraging words. He looked from Carol to Michael.

"Hey good buddy," he said. Then Chris looked at Mark.

"Everything is okay, Chris," Mark said. I asked for someone to get Patrick and Mark left the room. Chris' eyes widened as he watched his oldest brother leave.

"It's okay, sweetheart. Mark is getting Patrick," I told him. He calmed down to show that he understood. He glanced over at Poppa Bob.

"Good to see you buddy," Poppa said with tears in his eyes.

"Hey Chris," Pat said, walking in the room. Chris smiled and tried to talk. It had been several days since he had last spoken and I was thrilled to hear his voice again. He looked at each one of us, taking his time saying something that sounded like "Ma."

I turned to Mark, "Is he trying to say 'Mom'?" I asked, but no one was sure.

"Chris, everything is okay. We're here for you. It's okay brother," Mark told him. Chris looked at each of us again from Poppa to Mark to Patrick to Michael to Carol, and finally back to me, smiling sweetly again, then he closed his eyes.

The air was still. I think everyone held their breath at the same time waiting for what would happen next, wondering, I'm sure, if Chris' time had come and if this was our last moment with him. I thought if he was trying to say "mom" if it meant that his mother was somehow with him. I had no idea how many minutes passed, but Chris' breathing never slowed and his heart continued its strong beats.

"Well, I guess Chris just wanted a midnight rally," Carol said.

"You are truly amazing," I whispered. I kissed his lips again and replaced the breathing tubes.

I prayed thanksgiving to God for this most incredible and loving moment with Chris. I was reminded that God is our Light even at midnight.

Chris wasn't ready to let go yet, and I had no idea what was going to happen or if he was waiting for something. But I knew one thing for sure – when Chris was ready, Jesus would shine His Light on the road for Chris to ride on home to Him.

Not Giving Up!

"I'm running hard for the finish line. I'm giving it everything I've got."
                                                              - 1 Corinthians 9:26

Where I fell asleep was exactly where I awoke the next morning, with my head on Chris' shoulder still holding his hand. I wondered what this new day would bring and thanked God for another day with my husband.

After Terry checked Chris' vitals and the morphine pump, I told her about our "Midnight Rally".

"What is he waiting for, Stephanie? Is there someone he could be holding on for?" I shook my head. Everyone close to him had seen him over the last several weeks. I couldn't think of anyone.

With a heavy heart, I asked Terry, "Do you think maybe Chris doesn't want me in here when he lets go?" She looked over at Chris and I saw him nod one time. Terry came around the bed to embrace me,

"Steph, I think we just got our answer about what he wants." I pushed her away.

"I can't believe he wouldn't want me in here," I hissed. "That doesn't sound like him. He has always wanted me by his side. I can't believe..." I cried. I sat there for a long time, wrestling on what to do and finally relented. If this was what Chris wanted, then I would respect and honor him for it, even though it was breaking my heart.

"If this is what you want Chris, I'll support you." I choked. I kissed his forehead, his cheeks, and finally his lips.

"I love you," I whispered one more time.

Just before I reached the doorway, I looked at my husband for what I believed to be the last time. It took every bit of strength and courage I had to turn around and walk out of our bedroom.

When I reached the dining room, Carol immediately came to my side and helped me sit down. I told her, Poppa, and Chris' brothers what had just happened, sobbing uncontrollably. They couldn't believe it would be what Chris wanted and tried to comfort me. Terry came out, sat across from me, and held my hand.

"I asked Chris if it was better for him that you're not in the room when he lets go, and he nodded again. I'm so sorry, Stephanie," Terry whispered.

I begged everyone to stay close by him for me. I stayed at the table and wrestled with my promise to always be with Chris and his wish that I not be next to him. The pain in my heart, in my mind, and in my body was more than I could bear. I prayed.

"Anyone who is having troubles should pray! If you lack wisdom, ask God and it will be given to you."

- James 5:13 and 1:5

For the rest of the morning, I watched everyone enter and leave my bedroom, anxious to know what was happening which was the same answer, "He's calm." The pain of being away from my husband was so agonizing, I stood just outside my bedroom, hoping somehow Chris could feel my presence there just as strongly as if I was next to him on the bed. Each time someone found me there, I was guided back to my chair in the dining room and comforted once more. Teddie Momma came and stayed close by me, holding my hand. Like the others, she couldn't believe Chris would want this. I laid my head down on the table, not knowing how much more I could take and we prayed for guidance and strength.

"Fear not, I am with you; I am your God. I will give you strength. I will bring you help."

- Isaiah 41:10

The next thing I knew, I felt a warm, gentle squeeze on my shoulder. I opened my eyes and saw Father Don looking down at me. I was so relieved to see him, but I had no energy to move. He sat next to me and listened to me.

"Stephanie, what is your heart telling you to do right now?"

"I want to be with my husband," I exclaimed, "but he doesn't want me there. I saw him nod, Father. Even though this is the hardest thing I've ever done, but if this is what he wants, I have to respect him."

In his quiet demeanor, Father Don smiled, squeezing my hand.

"Oh, the love you have for Chris to stay out here knowing it's breaking your heart to do it. But, Stephanie, I can't believe for one second that he would not want you by his side. Knowing the two of you, how much you love each other, and seeing the two of you together, I can't believe that at all. So, let me ask you again," and he pointed to my chest, "what is your heart telling you to do?"

"My heart is telling me to be with Chris."

"Then why are you still sitting here?"

I jumped out of my chair so fast that it fell over. Before I entered the hallway to our bedroom, I turned around. "Father, will you come with me?"

I walked quietly into my bedroom. "I'm so sorry, Chris. I'm never leaving your side again. I thought I was doing what you wanted me to do. I love you so much." I kissed his cheek, sat down in the chair next to him, took his hand and stroked my cheek the way he used to.

"Steph, what are you thinking about right now?"

"The way Chris used to touch my cheek. I love how his hands feel against my face. We always held hands. It was one of the ways that kept us close."

Suddenly, Chris started grunting and moaning, shaking his head side to side. I stood up and started massaging his forehead, hoping to calm him down as Father Don walked around to the other side of the bed and held his hand.

"Chris, it's Father Don and I'm here with you and Stephanie. It's okay, Chris."

Chris moaned louder. He started punching the bed and thrashed his head back and forth violently. He sat up suddenly and began punching the air. Carol rushed into the room to see what was going on and pulled me away from Chris.

"Get out of here, Steph. You don't need to see this." Paralyzed with fear, I couldn't move. "Go! Father Don and I will calm Chris down."

I turned around and ran into Poppa's arms. He held me tightly as I sobbed.

"Why? What is going on today? They said it would be peaceful. That's not my husband in there. He's not peaceful. Why can't it be peaceful for him?" I cried, pounding on Poppa's back. He held me until my knees weakened and then helped me to a chair to sit down.

"My flesh and my heart may fail, but God is the strength of my heart."

- Psalm 73:26

I saw Father Don at the table and he told me Chris had calmed down and Carol was with him. I laid my head down on the table, feeling completely spent. Eventually Carol came out and told me it was okay to be with Chris.

"What happened?" I asked, but she didn't know and offered to call Terry to find out what we could do for him. I let her take over so I could be with Chris.

"I'm here, Chris," I whispered in his ear. "I'm here. I love you so much." His skin felt like it was on fire. When Mark, Patrick, and Michael came in, I asked them about it. They told me Carol was talking to hospice on the phone. Mark massaged Chris' feet while I continued to massage his forehead and eyebrows. Michael wiped Chris' face with a damp, cool washcloth while Patrick kept an eye on the morphine pump. We worked together silently in the best way we knew how to comfort Chris. Carol told us that Dr. Needles was ordering another pump to intravenously give Chris the Ativan rather than trying to give it to him orally.

Several hours later, the pharmacy delivery showed up with an extra pump and Ativan. A different hospice nurse came, but she didn't know how to connect the second pump. I looked at her exasperated – Chris needed this now. Carol offered to show her since she was certified as a nurse practitioner. I gave the nurse permission to allow my sister to help, waiving her from any responsibility and liability. But she insisted that it had to be a hospice nurse. Carol titled her head toward the door for me to leave. Frustrated, I walked into the dining room and fell into a chair next to Teddie Momma. I laid my head down and she stroked my hair, helping me calm down.

Out of the blue, Poppa suggested playing Scrabble. Everyone agreed and he set up the board game. In no time, we started joking and laughing, challenging each other. It seemed like all the anxiety, stress, and tension of the day disappeared in a friendly competition over words. I knew Chris would've liked this.

An hour later, a knock came from the door and I ran to open it. Seeing it was Terry who had come to help, I hugged her feeling so relieved my husband would get the kind of care he needed.

After another hour, Chris seemed more subdued and we knew the Ativan pump was working for him. Feeling relieved and exhausted, I carefully climbed onto the bed next to my husband and fell asleep on his shoulder. According to Carol and Chris' brothers, we slept peacefully throughout the night.

"Be still and know that I am God"

- Psalm 48:15

The Finish Line:
Thursday, January 29, 2009

"I have fought the good fight."

- 1st Timothy 4:7

I woke up early with the sun shining on my face. I lifted my head to check on Chris and he was still fighting strong. I admired his perseverance while wondering what he was waiting for.

"Good morning," I whispered. "Today is a good day." I couldn't get enough of looking at my husband. Even though Chris was unable to speak or move, I felt his love for me at that moment more than the day he first said those beautiful words to me. I don't know how to explain it, but there was a sense of joy and peace within me. I thanked God again for blessing us with each other. We would have missed out on an incredible experience of love if we had never met. I truly believed God's Hand was on us and we had fulfilled His plan together.

"I believe God brought us together for a reason. I believe the day we met, our lives were being blessed. I believe God brought us close so I can cherish you, share what's most important to your heart and to always love you."

- Author Unknown

Later in the morning, Teddie Momma came and presented me with a gift that had arrived at her house late yesterday afternoon. She told me a story about a group in her friend's church in Massachusetts who pray for certain people while knitting a shawl together. I opened the box, closed my eyes and let my fingers explore the soft yarn. I've never felt yarn as soft as this shawl felt to me. I opened my eyes, pulling the shawl out of the box. The colors resembled the fall leaves perfectly: brown, green, red, and orange with specks of gold. I wrapped it around my shoulders and immediately felt the warmth of its love and the power of its prayer. I hugged Teddie Momma thanking her for this precious gift and went in to share it with Chris. I described the shawl and the purpose of it as I brushed it on his hands, arms, and cheeks. I was amazed how people we didn't know had taken the time to pray for us while making this shawl. I talked to Chris about how people in different states were thinking of us and praying for us. I reminded him that we were blessed in so many ways.

Early in the afternoon, I found out Michael had an emergency and needed to return home to take care of it so I gave him some time alone with Chris. He read scriptures from Psalm 23 and 27, Isaiah 40, and Ephesians 6 encouraging Chris to know God was with him just as we all were.

The day continued with such a surreal kind of peace, one that I cannot explain except through this scripture:

"... and the peace of God, which surpasses all understanding, will keep your hearts and minds in Christ Jesus."

- Philippians 4:7

I played classical music with the soft rain in the background, knowing how much Chris enjoyed it and how it helped him relax.

"Oh Chris, do you know how much I adore you? How much I love you? Do you know how much your smile lights up the room and seems to make all the problems go away? Do you know how much it means to me when you say or do something so thoughtful and totally unexpected at a moment when I need it most? Do you know how much pride I hold in my heart for the kind of man you are – for your strength, your gentleness, your courage, your faith, your love, and your hope? Do you know how much I need you by my side in the best of times, in the worst of times, and in all the times in between? Chris, it never mattered to me where we were or what we were doing, what mattered most was that you and I were together and loving each other through it all. Oh sweetheart, I know you'll always watch over me and be with me all the days of my life. I love you more than words can express."

I was interrupted with a phone call from Father Don who called to check how things were going. I told him about the prayer shawl and the peacefulness of the day. It was so good to hear his voice and he shared a special prayer that added to the peace I felt in my heart.

Late in the afternoon, Carol pulled me close to her.

"Steph, I don't think it's going to be much longer. Spend every minute with Chris." I looked at her completely stunned. I'd been through this several times from Terry, but my sister has never uttered these words to me.

"Really? Are you sure?" With tears in her eyes, she nodded and hugged me tightly.

Suddenly, I felt a panic overwhelm me. "Bob!" I exclaimed. "I need to find him and get him here." I rushed to the phone and called his house – no answer. I called his gym – Bob wasn't there. I called his cell phone – no answer. Finally, I called Kelly's cell phone – no answer. I didn't know what else to do, so I lifted my hands up and prayed.

God, you know Bob needs to be here. Please, get him here. Bless these two best friends with one more moment together.

I went back to Chris and draped our shawl over the both of us to calm down and feel that peace again.

The ringing of the phone broke the silence and I jumped up to answer it, hoping it was Bob. It was Kelly apologizing for not having her cell phone with her.

"Kelly," I interrupted, "where's Bob? What is he doing right now?"

"He's getting ready for work tonight."

"Kelly, Bob needs to be here. *Now.* Can you get him here?"

"Let me call you back, Stephanie." 10 minutes later, she told me they were on their way.

Thank you, God. Somehow I knew everything was going to be okay.

"Chris," I whispered, getting back in bed next to him, "Bob is on his way."

The sun slowly dropped below the horizon and the stars brilliantly lit up the night sky – adding to the serenity of the day. Patrick continued to monitor the morphine pump while talking quietly with Mark and Talal, Carol's husband. When Bob walked in, I got up quickly and hugged him.

"Bob, you're supposed to be here. Thank you, Kelly, for getting him here." I asked if he wanted to be alone with Chris and he shook his head.

"No. I want you all to stay here too." I watched Bob tenderly take his best friend's hand and whispered in Chris' ear for a few minutes. Kelly came over to the other side of the bed to sit by me. Then Bob sat in the chair next to Chris, still holding his hand, and started telling stories that made us laugh. Chris would have loved this since he always enjoyed a funny story.

A half-an-hour later, Bob checked his watch and slowly rose from his chair, regrettably telling us he had to leave for work. He leaned over to Chris one last time and said goodbye. He paused several times to look at his best friend before he finally left.

I settled down next to Chris and noticed a change in his breaths. He was taking in longer gasps, breathing slower. Mark immediately joined Patrick at Chris' side and Talal went to get Carol. When she walked in, she took one look at Chris and nodded. But I didn't need her confirmation. I already knew what was happening.

"I have fought the good fight, I have finished the race."

- 2nd Timothy 4:7 – 8

I wrapped my arms around my husband.

"Chris, I will love you all the days of my life," I whispered. "Thank you for loving me. Go home to Jesus. I love you, Chris. I love you. I love you..."

After 20 short minutes, Chris took his final breath. There was a still silence in the room. With my sister embracing me, Mark and Patrick close by their brother, Talal patting his feet, Teddie Momma whispering prayers over us, Poppa Bob and Momma Sue looking over the man who became their son, and even little Bridget resting her head on Chris' leg, we said our own goodbye, letting him go.

I don't know how much time had passed, but when I looked up, I saw Bob and Kelly tearfully walked back into the bedroom.

"Bob, Chris was waiting for you!" I cried out to him. "The other night, we thought he was saying 'Mom' but he was trying to say *your* name, 'Bob.' He needed his best friend and you came."

Chris was waiting for Bob, his riding partner, to help him cross over his finish line victoriously.

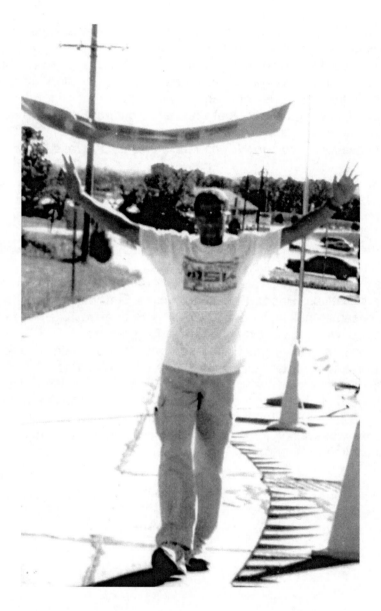

"I pressed on 'till I possessed Christ Jesus. I raced forward and ran toward the goal, my eyes on the prize to which God has called me from above in Christ Jesus."

— Philippians 3:12, 13, 14

Epilogue

Six weeks later, I was at Bob and Kelly's house seeking their comfort during one of the darkest days of my life. The pain of missing my husband was so unbearable, I couldn't stand to be alone in my grief. Through my sobs, I asked Bob if he would tell me what he told Chris that finally made him ready to let go. Bob nodded.

"Steph, I said, 'Chris, I want you to know that I'll be watching over Stephanie. You don't need to worry, she'll be well taken care of. I love you, good buddy, but it's time.' Then I prayed the 'Our Father' knowing it would help him be at peace."

I will always be grateful to Bob for sharing his last words to his best friend with me. He didn't have to, but out of his love for Chris and me, he did.

Again, God showed me how His love will always light our darkest moments. It was through this act of love between two best friends and from my husband that I began to heal in my grief.

Chris persevered in his faith, hope, and love as he endured the most challenging race of his life. He had cancer, but it never could destroy his spirit. His purpose here was complete, he rode in his race well, and he was victorious.

"We know that in everything God works for the good of those who love Him, whom He has called according to His plan."

-Romans 8:28

Now it is up to me to continue on in my race and I *will* ride on.

It is also up to you – will you ride on?

Whatever it is you're going through, no matter how rough the road, remember you're not alone. God is right there with you. Don't give up. Stay on the course. Grow deeper in your faith and trust God to be with you through it. Let hope give you the strength to keep going. Love each other through the race and you will be victorious through Christ Jesus.

"Since we are surrounded by such a great cloud of witnesses,
let us throw off everything that hinders
and let us run with perseverance the race marked out for us.
Let us look to Jesus the founder of our faith,
who will bring it to completion."

Hebrews 12:1, 2

Ride On!

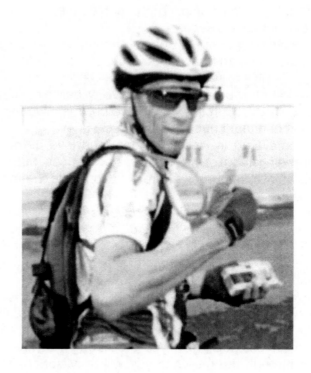

CPSIA information can be obtained at www.ICGtesting.com
Printed in the USA
LVOW101147250912

300244LV00001B/4/P